MW01716170

Excerpts from reviews:

"*Meeting the Challenge* isn't a typical 'When life hands you a lemon, make lemonade' self-help book. The author, Audrey Kron, a medical psychotherapist and licensed marriage counselor, really understands what the word 'challenge' means. The topics Kron has chosen to include in *Meeting the Challenge* are universal to all chronic illnesses, including psoriasis. The story of how Kron was able to get herself out of bed each day and put one foot in front of the other to get where she is, can inspire others to take stock of what is important in their lives and learn how to capitalize on positive things."

Susan Terry,
National Psoriasis Foundation

"*Meeting the Challenge* --- is destined to become a classic reference on down-to-earth, practical suggestions for coping with a variety of issues. As with her first book, Audrey's writing style is clear, comfortable, and easily read. It is like a conversation with a well-trusted, empathic friend who knows us and responds to us personally out of her own experience. Each topic is introduced with a letter from a reader with a specific question about managing chronic illness, to which Audrey responds with several suggestions for coping, along with a hearty dose of encouragement and the assurance that we are not alone in our thoughts, feelings, or experiences."

Judy Sobezak, Ph.D.,
Michigan Women Psychologist Network

"*Meeting the Challenge*: *Living with Chronic Illness* is a down-to-earth guide that is highly useful to many people. It is reaffirming to readers who experience a range of emotions and encounter a variety of challenges in dealing with their own chronic illness or the illness of a loved one. *Meeting the Challenge* provides practical guidance that really will help people persevere in the face of a major health challenge."

Jeff Crowley, Associate Executive Director,
National Association of People with AIDS

"This book is filled with educational, practical, sometimes humorous and always sensitive affirming suggestions for coping with chronic illness from both the patient and family perspective. Throughout the book, Audrey takes every opportunity to empower her reader and is able in a very credible way to offer suggestions for coping that make sense. Solutions to problems range from how to deal with doctors, friends and family, to coping with disappointment and recurrence. As a social worker and EAP counselor, I value her efforts and find the book invaluable as a resource for my clients."

Mary Ellen Gaffney, MSW, EAP,
Hutzel Hospital, Detroit, Michigan

“Ms. Kron gives her readers a wealth of information and insight into living well in spite of chronic illness. She is well qualified to write on the topic. Ms. Kron is a medical psychotherapist and licensed marriage counselor specializing in working with people affected by chronic illness. Her interest in the topic is more than academic, though. She has had to deal with numerous health crises and surgeries. She has done so with grace and courage, and through it all she has been a wife, a mother, a student, a community activist and a respected professional.”

Celia Savonen, Social Worker
Myasthenia Gravis Association,
Detroit Chapter

“This book is like a road map for persons who don't know where to start when learning how to cope with a chronic illness. The book is an upbeat, inspiring guide to those with chronic illness. As Kron positively asserts, ‘By using our coping skills, we can meet the challenge’.”

Debbie Adams Roraback, MSW,
Chronic Illness Awareness Coalition

“Reading Audrey Kron's second book *Meeting the Challenge: Living with Chronic Illness* is like reading an owner's manual for a car needing maintenance and repair. Audrey has combined the ‘nuts and bolts’ how-to advice of a fellow chronic illness patient with a professional's view of dealing with emotions, relationships, stress, and a family member's perspective. Whether you are just beginning, or an ‘old pro’ at dealing with chronic illness, you will learn from this travel guide for people living with pain, uncertainty and unending challenge.”

Don Young, HPN Consumer,
President of The Oley Foundation, Crohn's patient

“After reading the story of Audrey's life, it's clear that she is someone who believes in Margaret Mead's declaration that ‘one person can make a difference’. The book includes Audrey's inspiring personal story and practical suggestions for dealing with chronic illness. There are also chapters on relationships, psychological issues, and specific coping techniques plus chapters written by Audrey's husband, Lawrence Kron, discussing Chronic Illness from a family member's perspective.”

Rebecca Chalker,
Interstitial Cystitis Association

“The book addresses difficult issues, such as sexuality and incontinence, with honesty and compassion. Kron's sympathetic approach and sound advice make it a helpful resource for anyone living with Crohn's disease, ulcerative colitis, or any other chronic illness.”

Crohn's Colitis Foundation of America

"Her approach is gentle and understanding and often left me feeling as if she was actually in the room talking with me. At the same time, she does not let the reader forget that continually feeling sorry for ourselves will get us nowhere. Areas which have been of ongoing difficulty for me, which I had not found addressed in other books, were dealt with here."

Alice Morgan,
Michigan Parkinson Diseases Association

"I read your book with great interest, and I feel that you should be complimented for your good work. As a long term sufferer, I look at your work and I think that you have excellent intuition, and dispense good advice. I feel there are some excellent analogies, and that RSD patients can benefit from these. Most beneficial are the explanations on 'handling things' such as career, family, etc."

Francis J. Davis, Jr., Director,
Reflex Sympathetic Dystrophy Syndrome Association

"---this book does not center on a specific illness; the information provided is useful for people with any chronic illness and their loved ones. The book uses mostly a question-and-answer format and presents information in an easily-accessible format interspersed with experiential accounts and humor, including cartoons. The book also assumes no prior knowledge and explains in detail what many would wrongly assume that everyone knows—such as what to bring to the hospital for patients and visitors, and exactly what happens when you go in for a procedure. The author provides a very comprehensive list of groups and organizations which includes name, address, phone, fax, e-mail and web site information, plus a large reading list. We would recommend this book as an easy-to - use reference guide to anyone with a chronic illness."

Rosa Bustamanta, volunteer,
Diane Lynch, student intern
National Multiple Sclerosis Society

"Choosing a doctor, dealing with pain, travel, work, getting up in the morning, handling recurrences, finding a spouse, relationships, sexual matters, embarrassment, coping, dealing with stress, being a good visitor and thoughts on happiness comprise some of the wide range of topics making this book a must for anyone living with a chronic illness, their loved ones, or professionals working with them. Extensive information on readings, support groups, and chapters on the family perspective, written by Audrey's husband who is a psychologist, are also included."

Fibromyalgia Resources

"*Meeting the Challenge: Living with Chronic Illness* speaks to all of us who either has a chronic illness or lives with someone who does. Some days the sun shines, and other days it doesn't. Audrey has written about how to cope with the ups and downs of dealing with a chronic illness and gives some wonderfully practical advice that sometimes get overlooked when we talk to other individuals who are dealing with chronic illness. Thank you Audrey for putting into words what so many of us feel."

Vicky Holets Whittemore, Ph.D.,
Vice President for Medical and Scientific Affairs,
National Tuberous Sclerosis Association

"*Meeting the Challenge* is a practical, helpful approach to individuals faced with every-day challenges. It provides strength and inspiration for the consumer, their families and friends, and is authored in an 'easy to read' fashion. Anyone living with a chronic illness has many topics to reference that inspire and focus on what is important for living a quality life. I commend Audrey Kron, M.A., C.G.P., for her courage, honesty and compassion and for taking the lead by sharing her experiences that are so helpful to others."

Lynda K. Anderson
President and Chief Operating Officer,
Sickle Cell Disease Association of America, Inc.

Meeting the Challenge

Living with Chronic Illness

by Audrey Kron M.A., CGP
Author of *Ask Audrey*

Meeting the Challenge

ISBN: # 0-9633877-1-5

Printed in the United States of America

Layout & Design by Elizabeth Pernick

Cover design by Doug Braunschweig

This printing was supported by a generous contribution from Hoechst Marion Roussel.

Second printing

This book was printed using recycled paper.

To my courageous patients
who continually teach me
new ways of meeting the challenge.

ACKNOWLEDGMENTS

Writing a book like this has been a challenge for me. However, it would not have been possible without the wonderful support I received. Words are not adequate to express my appreciation to the many people that helped make *Meeting the Challenge* a reality.

However, I want to sincerely acknowledge the following people:

My husband, Larry, who has been there for me in countless ways. He always says that he doesn't need acknowledgment, but it makes me feel better to let him know how much he's appreciated.

Edith Broida, my editor and dear friend. Edie spent hours reading, editing, rereading. Her encouragement kept me going. Not only is Edie a fine editor, but she defines the word friendship.

My family, for their love, patience and understanding. They have lived through the difficult days with me and have been so thrilled to see it all finally having a purpose.

My literature group and all my other wonderful friends who have brought me chicken soup and love, and were an important part of my motivation to keep going. Special friends are the best medicine one can have.

Elizabeth Pernick, who helped me with the technical aspects of laying out the book. Betty helped me get the book into my computer and then was there for all the emergencies that came up as I struggled with my computer skills. A special thanks to her sons Rob and Neal, who walked us through some difficult computer moments.

Dr. Jason Bodzin and Dr. Everette Rottenberg, who not only read the book for medical accuracy, but are important members of my medical team.

Robert Kron for contributing his time and talent to create the cartoons for *Meeting the Challenge.*

Elaine Yaker, who used her photographic skill to get the picture I needed. Not only was she talented, but she also was able to work fast enough to meet the deadline.

The following people who diligently went over each word and idea. A special thanks to Marion Cashero, Tracy Grossman, Dr. Rena Gordon, Joyce Kaplan, Ilene Karson, Esther Liwazer, Elizabeth Liwazer, Donna Ryan, Dr. Laurence Spickler, Ilene Wolosin and Sharon Zamezyk.

Dr. Marsha Vannicelli, who came from Boston to help with finishing touches. Her friendship and expertise as an author and therapist are greatly appreciated.

I'm grateful to Dr. John Gray, Dr. Paul Pearsall, Sefra Kobrin Pitzele, Virginia Ladd, Betty Sheldon, Dr. Bernie Siegel, and Alan Spoon who took time out of their busy lives to review the book.

Most of all, my clients, people who called and wrote letters, and all the individuals and family members struggling with a chronic illness. The courage and perseverance they have shown have been an inspiration to me.

PREFACE

Dear Readers,

Many of you may have already read my first book, *Ask Audrey*. That book was designed mainly for people with inflammatory bowel disease (IBD) and their families. It has been gratifying to receive so many comments, cards and letters assuring me that the book had been helpful to IBD patients and their families. What I hadn't expected though, was that the book would also satisfy some of the needs of people with other chronic illnesses. They welcomed the guidance *Ask Audrey* offered.

This book is written in response to the questions I received from those who have other chronic diseases. When I originally became a medical psychotherapist, I specialized in clients with inflammatory bowel disease. However, I was soon asked to work with people suffering from other illnesses. I quickly learned that each illness has its own particular features, but all share many common issues. The topics I have chosen to address in this book are universal to all illnesses. The questions are the actual questions I received in my "Ask Audrey" columns in the newsletters for the Chronic Illnesses Awareness Coalition, and the Crohn's Colitis Foundation of America, Michigan Chapter. In some cases they are composites of frequently asked questions I have encountered in my psychotherapy practice.

I have addressed issues for individuals and family members in all stages of illness. This book is not designed for a single reading. It should be retained as a reference for the many challenges that chronic illness presents. Therefore, I have designed *Meeting the Challenge* so that each chapter can be read independently. This will enable you to return to individual chapters as needed. However, in order to accomplish this, sometimes information is repeated. Hopefully, this will reinforce some of the more helpful ideas. Occasionally, I have referred to another section to add to a topic. The overall format should prove easy to follow.

Those of you who have read *Ask Audrey* will notice some of the ideas presented here appeared in that book. After great deliberation, I decided certain material was important to complete my story. Some coping techniques apply to all chronic illnesses, and I want to share them with my new readers. Much more has been added for the wider audience this book will reach.

Again I have left room for notes and encourage you to add your own ideas to personalize this book. We often lose track of valuable ideas during difficult bouts of our illness. Recording them here will enable you to keep a convenient record of your medical history, feelings, and thoughts, in one handy place.

Having a chronic illness is a "family affair." My husband, Lawrence Kron, Ph.D., has added a chapter regarding the family's perspective. Rather than reading what pertains to them, I suggest that family members and patients read the entire book. That way, family members will profit by having a better understanding of their loved ones who suffer from a chronic illness. We, in turn, can benefit from trying to understand what our families are experiencing.

This book is not a medical text. The coping skills I mention are ones that I have found to be effective. Most of the information I am sharing with you comes from working with clients who have chronic illness, as well as my own experience of living with it. I have consulted with many other professionals, as well as individuals with different illnesses, to convey as accurate a picture as possible. Still, not every answer will apply to you. Each case is different. However, I hope by the time you finish this book, you will have a repertoire of coping skills to help improve the quality of your life.

As always, I welcome your feedback or questions. If you have found something particularly helpful or if you have ideas to share, perhaps I can include them in the next book.

You may reach me at the address or phone number listed at the back of the book.

Dare to Dream with Greatness

When you dare to dream,
Dare to dream with greatness.
But when you dream great things,
Be prepared for a great adventure.

Many times you will need great courage;
More than you may think you truly possess.
But if you do what you believe in your heart,
Your courage will rise to meet your need.

Along the way others may not understand
But they will come to respect you for trying.
At times, you may not understand yourself.
But hold to your dreams and follow your heart.

You may not always succeed. But sometimes,
Just trying is as much of an accomplishment.
For success is made from both wins and losses,
And it does matter how you play the game.

True success is measured in small steps.
In numerous but small, personal victories.
In having a dream and working toward it.
In making even a small difference in your world.

Reaching for greatness takes very little daring.
The greater risk in life is to never even try.
It is more satisfying to say, "I tried but didn't win."
Rather than ask yourself, "What if I had tried?"

So when you dream, dream with greatness
And you will discover an even sweeter success.
You will discover the greatness others see in you
And a wonderful greatness within yourself.

— by R. S. Zate 1994

CONTENTS

Chapter One

MORE OF MY STORY

HERE WE GO AGAIN

At six o'clock on a cold morning in March 1994, I awoke to go to the bathroom. Something was not right. I felt very dizzy and fell back in bed. I was nauseated and the room was spinning. Somehow, I woke my husband and spoke urgently; "Larry, I need to get to the hospital!" Seeing the state I was in, he replied that he would carry me to the car. But I was terrified, and cried out that I couldn't be moved. "Call 911," was all I could gasp.

A few days earlier I had read a magazine article on healthy living, which caused me to reflect on my present lifestyle. Actually, it was a happy time. I was very satisfied with my career as a medical psychotherapist and marriage counselor. I had even decided that my experience of living with Crohn's disease from the time I was sixteen had strengthened my ability to counsel others. I had experienced many hospital stays and surgeries, which left me without an appendix, a uterus, a colon, most of my ileum, and most recently, the development of "sluggish" kidneys. Nevertheless, I felt my experience with illness had not been in vain.

My first book, *Ask Audrey*, was now in its third printing. I had heard from readers all over the world! Still, the article on healthy living made me realize I was deficient in one area: exercise. To remedy that, I had resolved that I would walk aerobically through the halls of Hutzel Hospital in Detroit (where I was on staff) whenever I had a break between clients.

While going down the stairs a few days earlier, in the midst of a brisk walk, I fell and hit my head with a real thud. Twenty people appeared from nowhere as I lay on the landing, too stunned to move. I was taken to the emergency room, then to the employee health office, and finally to the x-ray department. Afterwards, I returned to work. The doctor said that I seemed all right, but warned if I became nauseated or dizzy, or if there was any difficulty rousing me, it could be an indication of concussion and I should be taken straight to the hospital.

In all my years of going to the hospital, I had never called "911" or used an ambulance. There had been many emergencies, but I always had time to grab a few items and to be taken by car. Sometimes I even drove myself. This time was a totally new experience.

The EMS squad arrived quickly and set to work, trying to assess the state of my condition. With them were members of both the police and fire departments. I knew I was desperately sick when I didn't even bother with a robe or coat. It had snowed again, and you could feel the chill in the air. We had been having a particularly difficult winter.

The EMS crew wrapped me in a blanket and gently eased me onto the stretcher. It seemed as if I was at an amusement park, but this time there was no cotton candy. I had chills and yet was burning up. I couldn't stop vomiting, and I still had the terrible sensation of falling and spinning around. At first I thought I was dying. Then, it suddenly occurred to me that I might have some type of brain damage as a result of my fall at Hutzel.

I didn't even want to think of where that might lead. The EMS technician was trying to calm me, saying it was probably just a virus. As a psychotherapist, I knew what he was doing. I was afraid the situation was very serious and he needed somehow to ease my anxiety and to reassure me.

We sped through the early morning traffic to the emergency room. The ride seemed to last forever. At the hospital the doctors weren't sure if I was suffering from an infection or head injury. I should explain that as a result of the many intestinal operations I have had over the years, I was left with 'short gut syndrome' which necessitates total parenteral nutrition, also known as TPN. The TPN requires the insertion of a port under my skin. This port serves as an access to receive intravenous feeding six nights a week. The biggest problem with having a port is the tendency to develop infections. At various times my port has been replaced because of the infections.

The previous August, for example, I had developed a staph infection, and nothing seemed to alleviate it. Ultimately, the port had been removed and a new one inserted—a difficult procedure, because all the veins in my chest had dried up. However, my physician, Dr. Jason Bodzin, managed to find a vein in my leg and threaded the line all the way up to my chest.

Now, the doctors in the emergency room were concerned that the chills might indicate a new infection in the port. Another possibility was a head injury from the fall. The doctors weighed their choices and decided to start me on antibiotics, ordering tests to rule out any other problems. A few hours later, I was stabilized and admitted to the hospital.

By now, Larry had to leave for the office. Since we are both psychotherapists, we knew the importance of being there for our clients. I knew that I wouldn't be able to work that day and asked Larry to cancel my appointments. I had a meeting scheduled at our house that morning for my Temple's women's group, and I asked Larry to postpone that as well.

There was one more complication. Larry was 'opening' that night in a community theater production of "Prelude to a Kiss." He was cast in the role of the father of the bride, and it was his biggest part yet. Larry and I originally became involved in community theater because of our daughter Karen's interest in acting. There were no understudies for this show and I knew the whole cast was counting on him.

At first, I insisted he stay in the emergency room with me, even though the nurses tried to limit him to five minutes every hour. I knew I needed an advocate there. At one point, he told the nurses I was accustomed to hospitals, and familiar with pain, and that when I became distraught they should take it seriously and not just think I was hysterical or overly dramatic. Finally, the chills abated and I was left feeling just dizzy and miserable.

The orderlies then wheeled me up to room 2913. I tried to think of "13" as lucky but still felt superstitious about the number. I kissed Larry good-bye, dreading the rest of the day. It was already mid-afternoon. I had lots of time ahead of me—hopefully! I couldn't read because of my headache. I thought about calling my support people, but I didn't want to worry them. I still wasn't too sure what was happening. In retrospect, I should have made those calls. In reality, the phone wasn't working right, and I couldn't even hear incoming calls. The entire situation was extremely stressful. Yet I decided I would feel like a fraud if I couldn't overcome this latest challenge.

Fortunately, the television in the room was connected, and forcing my mind away from my body seemed like a good idea. I turned on the TV and tuned to "The Sonya Friedman Show." Much to my dismay, the topic that day was "How to Die." I definitely didn't want dying lessons. I fiddled with different channels and finally found Oprah Winfrey. She was interviewing a Holocaust survivor. At first, I doubted that would be helpful, but remembering the impact of "Schindler's List," motivated me to listen. The survivor related how he had been hidden in three yards of space with twelve other people, lying on top of each other, for **two years**! If they could do that, I decided I could be uncomfortable for one night. Thus, I managed until morning, and gradually the dizziness subsided. Though we never actually found out the cause, the symptoms eventually became minor and tolerable.

Soon after, I related this experience to my friend Connie Grossman, who responded, "Audrey, you really have to write about coping mechanisms." I had already been planning a second book on coping with chronic illness. However, it was easy to get sidetracked with my busy life. I managed to put the title on the refrigerator door, and periodically I jotted a few notes, but that was all. While I was still in the hospital, Edie Broida, my friend and editor for *Ask Audrey*, called to ask if I needed anything, since I had come so unprepared. I asked her for paper. The next day I sat up in bed with the lovely pad of pink lined paper she brought and started my second book, this time in earnest. I realized that this frightening experience in the hospital would be the beginning of this book: *Meeting the Challenge: Living With Chronic Illness.*

LOOKING BACK

Before continuing with the rest of my story, I would like to recount the beginnings of my experience with chronic illness for readers who have not read *Ask Audrey.*

I have few memories of being sick as a child. I do remember chicken pox. I sat on the front porch blowing bubbles out of a bubble pipe, and shared my toys. Soon the whole neighborhood had chicken pox.

At sixteen, I had my first experience in the hospital—an emergency appendectomy. I had no idea what to expect. On the way home, I told my father at least now I knew what to take with me if I ever returned. He just said, "Shhh," as if that would keep me from ever passing through the hospital doors again.

"Shhh," was not enough. That episode was just the beginning of many hospital stays. The hardest part of my appendix operation was trying not to laugh. Laughing hurt, and the frequent paging for what sounded like "Dr. Baked Beans" didn't help.

At seventeen, my health had not improved. Later, we realized the appendix operation was the result of a misdiagnosis. My high school drama teacher, Mr. White, was the first person to actually recognize how sick I was. He had cast me as Elizabeth Barrett in "The Barretts of Wimpole Street." Saying "Doctor, doctor," as I lay on the couch didn't require acting. Soon, I was in the hospital again for more testing. I never did get to play the role. Thirty years later, I was able to make up for that disappointment and take part in a production of "Fiddler on the Roof."

My medical tests in Detroit proved futile. The doctors still had no idea why I was in so much pain, and growing weaker all the time. They considered mononucleosis, but seemed tentative in their diagnosis. My family decided to make a pilgrimage to the Mayo Clinic.

In 1954 the Mayo Clinic was the mecca for any type of illness. People came from all over the world to find some hope. For many, it was the last resort. Most patients stayed in hotels, and scheduled various tests and treatments as outpatients. The restaurants in the area had become accustomed to seeing patrons with all kinds of medical problems. For example, one day I passed out at the table and without even blinking, the waitress brought a cold compress and continued to serve our table.

Before long, I was admitted to the hospital at Mayo because I was running a fever. That was an experience! Only the sickest were confined to the hospital. Because our insurance did not cover an out-of-state hospital, I decided against a semi-private room, and entered a twelve-bed ward. In the end bed lay Charlotte, who prayed aloud all day. Her body was encased in a neck-to-body cast, and she roller-skated in place to exercise her legs. Despite her own difficulties, she was quite supportive. Across the way was a country woman who kept a black satchel filled with food hidden under the bed. Periodically she would sneak under the bed for some forbidden nourishment. There was also Molly who wandered around with a bag of fluid hanging down, which was totally unfamiliar to me at that time. There were constant moans and screams. All in all, it wasn't an ideal vacation spot for anybody, let alone a seventeen-year-old.

Each day, the doctors would attempt some new diagnostic tool. One day I had to have a bone-marrow test. I already knew this had to do with leukemia. It was extremely painful. I had particular difficulty with this procedure because of a previous experience in Detroit. One intern asked, "Is this the right instrument to use?" My confidence was shattered. Later, I watched mothers in the waiting room preparing young children for what lay ahead. I still have a vivid picture of one mother talking to her son. He had looked so worried, but when the nurse called he lifted his head and just bravely marched in.

That night at Mayo, after the bone-marrow test, the intern stopped by my bed. I asked for the results. It was routine to tell me that each test was negative. This time the intern said in a solemn voice that they wanted to talk to my mother in the morning. I was convinced that I had a terminal illness.

Soon my mother arrived, but I didn't share my concern, and told her to go to the movies. I felt there was no sense in both of us worrying. That night I was sure I was going to die. I thought of how I wanted to spend my last days. The next morning, the doctors came and said they finally determined that I had ulcerative colitis. It was another misdiagnosis. Later they were to find out I had Crohn's disease, but I was so excited that I would live, I didn't care what I had.

Shortly after, I was discharged and we started the trip home. The long drive was difficult. I was so weak that I could hardly walk, let alone climb stairs. I also had terrible diarrhea, so we had to find restaurants with lavatories on the first floor. Because I was so sick, I would often just abandon my food and leave. To further complicate matters I had developed phlebitis because I had been so inactive in the hospital. On the way home, the pain was so intense that when we stopped at my Aunt Ethel and Uncle Bob's house, I couldn't be moved any further. The following week, just getting to the bathroom was an ordeal.

I continued to struggle with my illness and with difficulty, managed to graduate from high school. It wasn't that I had trouble with my studies, but I did have trouble with my lack of energy. Climbing stairs was overwhelming. In particular, I remember Miss Harnack. Everyone else thought she was mean, but often she would let me rest instead of going to class, and allowed me to stay upstairs during practice fire-drills.

When graduation day rolled around, everyone was worried about whether I would be able to walk across the stage to accept a scholarship award. I believe I was given a Chrysler scholarship because, by now, I had a deeper awareness of the meaning of life than most seventeen-year-olds did. I made it across the stage, but when the students marched out, I didn't have enough energy to go back with them.

Despite the illness, I became very involved in the B'nai B'rith Youth Organization. I served as chapter president, and then as Michigan regional president. When the election of officers took place, I had just had my appendix out and wasn't able to climb stairs. My best friend, Jeanie, found a young man to carry me up the stairs. The next day, both he and I were installed respectively as regional presidents for AZA and BBG (part of the B'nai B'rith Youth Organization). That's how I met Larry, the man who was later to become my husband.

Larry and I worked together in B.B.Y.O., and dated. Then he went off to the University of Michigan. During that time, and for years to come, there were frequent hospitalizations. During one such hospital stay, Larry came in for the weekend and visited me at the hospital. I suggested he date other girls, because I wasn't available for "normal" dating activities. He just said that as far as he was concerned, we were going steady. That was just the beginning of many times we would spend together in the hospital. More important though, it was the beginning of a marriage that is still going strong.

But I'm getting a little ahead of my story. I had been advised by my high school counselor not to go to college, because it would be too difficult physically. Nonetheless, with scholarship in hand, I registered at Wayne University (now Wayne State University). Again, just getting to and from class was harder than the classes themselves.

One day, I fell down in the snow and couldn't walk any farther. Some workmen picked me up and asked where I wanted to go. I pointed to my classroom and they brought me there. The teacher, who was becoming accustomed to my passing out, just said calmly, "Who wants to take Audrey home today?"

I became adept at planning around my illness. I knew if I got sick in the middle of the term, I could convince the teacher to let me make up the work. However, I knew that if I became sick in the beginning, it was hopeless. It would be impossible to start classes late. I also became quite an expert at negotiating with the "expediting committee." I had to schedule my classes based on their location. If they weren't close together, I knew I couldn't handle walking from one class to another.

Just getting to school was an ordeal. Without a car, it took me either 45 minutes on the bus, or else I arranged transportation. I remember feeling so weak, standing in the cold to catch a bus. But I still kept plugging away. During this period, I had my first intestinal surgery. At that time, medical practice dictated the early removal of inflamed sections of the intestine. Then, I believed, the surgery would eliminate the Crohn's disease.

Despite everything, Larry and I were married in 1956. Shortly after, we moved to Ann Arbor. Larry was already in law school, but I was still working on my undergraduate degree. I was proficient at finding classes according to location, but the Crohn's disease wasn't as easy to plan. The frequent hospitalizations slowed me down. I even tried taking correspondence courses one semester, when I couldn't manage getting to classes. As hard as I tried, I still wasn't done with my undergraduate work when Larry finished law school. I encountered endless red tape, but finally managed to finish my work at Wayne University and still earn my degree from the University of Michigan.

Larry landed a job in a Detroit law firm. At that time, beginning lawyers were asked if they had any additional income, since the wages were so low. We were happy to be receiving any income. As students, we were budgeting every last nickel. A Saturday night pizza was a big treat.

My degree was in education. I had wanted to be a psychiatrist, but most women at that time became teachers. It had been such a long struggle; I expected the bands to play, and the earth to stop for just a minute. However, since it had taken so long, there was no one I knew in my graduating class. So the news of my graduation came very unceremoniously, in a letter from the university. Inwardly, the bands did play, and I felt I had achieved a real victory. I was also five months pregnant.

Our son, Michael, made his debut at Sinai Hospital in Detroit. My obstetrician, Dr. David Feld, had been extremely cautious during my entire pregnancy. At one point, I wanted to go out on a boat, and he remarked dryly that I could — only if it was anchored! I couldn't really blame him. There was some question as to whether I should even get pregnant, and additional concerns about whether I could deliver a healthy baby. It had been decided I would have a Caesarean section. I was actually looking forward to it. I wanted, for once in my life, to walk into the hospital with my makeup on, my hair done, and wearing street clothes. I was accustomed to being rushed into emergency, when how I looked was my least concern.

As it turned out, Michael came earlier than expected. I didn't even realize I was in labor. I had been used to a lot of pain with the inflammatory bowel disease (IBD). I had heard women talking about labor pains, and expected this new pain would be much worse. Just in case, I did get out of bed and started folding laundry. When the pains were a few minutes apart, I woke Larry, and we called the doctor. He wanted me at the hospital immediately, so I still didn't get my dream fulfilled of going to the hospital "like a lady."

During Michael's early years, I was a wife and mother. I did volunteer work and took classes, but I felt I couldn't do anything that required a regular schedule. I was in the hospital so often, that Michael built hospitals instead of houses when he played with his blocks. At that time I kept a suitcase packed, since I had become a regular at Sinai Hospital. Larry once sent me a card addressed to "Audrey, Sinai Hospital, Detroit." With nothing more on the envelope it was delivered to me.

At this time, I developed a fistula, and nothing seemed to heal it. Dr. Frederick Coller, an Ann Arbor surgeon, suggested three surgeries to alleviate the problem. I had already been through several resections and was not looking forward to more surgery. I discussed the surgery with Dr. Meyer Teitelbaum, my internist.

Dr. Teitelbaum was a wonderful man. He has since died, but he was the epitome of what a doctor should be. He made me feel good the minute he entered my room. I called him my "booking agent." He was always willing to admit that someone else might have more information. Consequently, I came in contact with many wonderful doctors. Dr. Coller, who has also passed away, was among them. I had confidence in both of them, and went ahead with the triple surgery plan.

The first surgery was an ileostomy, (the diversion of fecal waste through a surgically created opening of the ileum to the body wall, enabling waste to be collected in an appliance attached to the skin by special adhesive). At that time there wasn't the information available that there is now. The ostomy group in Detroit was run by Tillie Bieman, a longtime ostomate who operated the only ostomy organization in Michigan from her home.

I'd like to be able to say that having the ostomy was a breeze. Years later, when I had my second ostomy, the situation was much different. But in those early years, it was a real struggle. Tillie was helpful in teaching me the mechanics. At that time there were no stoma therapists.

As soon as I was able, I became involved in the local ostomy group, and served as president for several years. In that capacity, I was instrumental in arranging a scholarship that enabled the first stoma therapist to be trained in Michigan. I dreamed of having a stoma therapist in every hospital, and today that dream is almost a reality.

I had the ostomy for about a year, and the next stage was to correct the fistula. The second operation accomplished this. Then the doctors wanted to eliminate the ostomy. By this time I had become used to it and questioned the decision, but I yielded to the medical opinions and the ostomy was reversed.

This turned out to make my life much worse. I had no control, and "accidents" became a way of life. In addition to the "accidents," I had to deal with the side effects of Prednisone, a drug that had become the new favored treatment for Crohn's disease. My condition did improve, but the resulting puffiness and the hair growth were difficult to accept. There was also the uncertainty of additional side effects.

During these years, I had been in the hospital more than thirty times. After thirty I stopped counting. There were times when I spent whole seasons in the hospital. I knew how they celebrated every holiday and what special treats I could expect on my dinner tray. Many times, we would rush to the emergency room. One time Larry asked the doctor when I would be able to come home, and he said, "Don't ask 'when,' ask 'if'."

Another time, I was suffering from an electrolyte imbalance and passed out. When I came to, I saw my family standing around the bed. I became alarmed when I saw my Uncle Harry. I knew he hated to come to the hospital. The first words out of my mouth were, "Uncle Harry's here. They think I'm dying." After that comment, I could never convince him that I understood his reluctance of coming to the hospital. He later became a frequent visitor.

Even the hospital staff were becoming accustomed to my frequent visits. I tried to keep my life as normal as possible, despite the interruptions. One resident physician, Bill Sills, came to my hospital room because he wanted to meet "the person who conducted bridge tournaments from her hospital bed." We didn't know it then, but later Bill, and his lovely wife, Michele, would become our very good friends.

I made a real effort to make my hospitalizations as pleasant as possible — a definite challenge. I decorated my room with pictures and cards. I established support systems with other patients and hospital staff. Finally, I tried to carry on my social life by inviting friends to visit, and arranging for refreshments. It was difficult, but possible. Granted, there were days when just turning over was a major endeavor. I just did the best I could.

During this time, my sister, Judie, was also diagnosed with Crohn's disease. Today we immediately consider IBD if a sibling presents gastrointestinal symptoms. However, at that time, she had to endure numerous tests to determine a diagnosis. I was out of town when she was finally hospitalized. As soon as I returned, I rushed right to the hospital. The first words out of her mouth were, "Audrey, you're a saint." I had no idea what she was talking about. She continued, "I used to visit you in the hospital, and you made it look like it was so much fun. It's not fun at all!" Subsequently, Judie too, learned how to make the most out of her bouts in the hospital.

Despite the constant difficulties with my illness, I still managed to be a wife and mother, do volunteer work, travel, work on a research team, play tournament bridge, and start a women's literature group. This group still continues as an important support system for me.

In the mid 1960s I had a miscarriage. During that period, many children needed homes. My husband and I decided to adopt. Bob, at age three months, became our second son. It was right after the assassinations of Robert Kennedy and Martin Luther King. Robert Martin Kron was named for both men, with the hope that his future would hold less violence.

Bob was an active child and there were days when I wondered if I had enough energy to last until Larry returned home from work. However, the love we had for each other and for our sons was so strong, that we decided we would adopt another child in a few years.

I was still the traditional wife and mother of our generation. But the world was starting to change. I had just read Betty Friedan's *Feminine Mystique* and was reading Germaine Greer's *The Female Eunuch* when Larry had to go out of town for a seminar. I decided that would be a good time to ask my single friend, Carol, over for dinner. She said that she was dating a new man and asked if Jim, a fellow social worker, could come as well. In my traditional view, I would have waited for Larry's return and then arranged to get together. However, with this new "liberation," I thought, "why not?" This may not seem like much now, but in those days we were very traditional.

At dinner that night, adoption became a topic of conversation. A short time later, Jim heard of a young mother who was looking for a good home for her baby, and so, once again, we became parents. This time it was a daughter, whom we named Karen Elizabeth.

With three children, and the many activities I was involved in, the years flew by. We continued to try to keep everything as normal as possible. I searched for ways to cope, with my limited energy, constant need for bathrooms, numerous doctor appointments, and frequent hospitalizations.

I gave up the presidency of the ostomy organization to encourage the growth of new leadership, and soon became involved in the National Foundation of Ileitis and Colitis (now called the Crohn's & Colitis Foundation of America). The Detroit group was just starting. We met in each other's homes, and started to build our dreams for the future. Many of those dreams have now been realized.

I became program vice-president, and was leading many of the meetings. Frequently, people would come up to me after the meeting, and ask for advice. I even started getting calls from others who were having difficulty living with IBD. Often I felt that I was doing therapy without a license. I toyed with the idea of going back to school, but it seemed formidable. Larry too, had thought of returning to school, and had become interested in a psychology program. He started classes immediately. It took me a semester to gather the courage to try.

I heard of a marriage counseling program at the University of Detroit. The program was highly regarded, but equally important to me was the convenient parking. All the classes and the clinic were then held in one building. It seemed like something I could handle.

Just filling out all the application forms seemed overwhelming. I saw an academic counselor, and was told that I would need some prerequisites before I was even eligible for the program. At first, I took just one class. Then I took two. Later I was able to handle a full course load. One day I looked around the classroom, and realized my fellow students were young enough to be my children. But I was so excited to be in school again, that was hardly a concern.

My health seemed to be holding up, and I managed the first year. However, at the end of that year, I was taking final exams when I noticed I was bleeding. I called Dr. Feld and he said "Cross your fingers, and cross your legs, and if it doesn't stop by tomorrow, come in." I took my final, but then had to see him the next day. He suspected cancer, and recommended some testing, and then possibly a hysterectomy.

For the second time, I thought my life might be over. I remember walking around taking in nature's beauty, and feeling even more sensitive to the love around me.

Everything in life seems to have a purpose. This period was no exception. We had become friendly with Harold Ogust who ran "Travel with Goren" Bridge cruises which Larry and I had taken from time to time. Harold had just been diagnosed with cancer, and would not see anybody. But I knew that he could not refuse to see me now. I didn't want to wait until there was a definite diagnosis. If I did not have cancer, he might refuse to see me, and if I did have cancer, I was afraid I wouldn't be able to travel. So Larry and I went off to New York to see Harold and his wife, Jean.

The tests came back positive. I was scheduled to have a hysterectomy. Fortunately, it was now summer vacation, and I would not miss any classes. After the hysterectomy, Dr. Feld was quite sure that they had removed all the cancer. Larry and I had planned a trip to France, and we set off. I saw the Louvre in a wheelchair, but by then that seemed to be an advantage rather than a disadvantage. We were able to travel with Harold and Jean, big "C" and little "c" for the cancer Harold and I had. Unfortunately, Harold wasn't as lucky as I was.

There was a new problem, however. While I had been in the hospital for the hysterectomy, the doctors found I had a kidney stone. Again, they wanted to operate. I promised that when I returned from France, I would take care of this, and I did. My travel schedule ended with a trip to the operating room.

Next on my agenda, was getting accepted into the marriage counseling program at the University of Detroit. Fifteen candidates were admitted each year, and many more applied. I was concerned that I would be rejected because I had a serious illness, and had spent so much time in the hospital. Yet, I didn't want to lie. What I did do, was turn how I had handled this illness into a convincing argument for my acceptance. This approach has served me well throughout the years.

I can't describe the excitement I felt when I learned I was accepted to the program. The next two years flew by. I had thought that I already knew a lot about psychology, but the new information seemed endless. If a professor digressed, it didn't matter to me. Everything was fascinating. One day, as I was intent on recording every word, I felt a gentle nudge. The student next to me was saying, "you don't have to take that down, Audrey. It won't be on the test." She didn't realize, my goals were much greater than having answers for a test.

During our group therapy course we were encouraged to conduct our own group. I was anxious to start a group for Crohn's and colitis patients. I asked Dr. Dick Spain, our group therapy teacher, to be my co-therapist. He was delighted to have a ready-made group, and I was happy to have someone with experience as a co-therapist.

The first group was very successful, and more followed. My husband, now working on his doctorate in psychology, joined me as a co-therapist for a couples' group dealing with IBD. We were all thrilled with our progress, and Dick suggested we submit our work for presentation. The International Group Psychotherapy Association accepted our paper, and we were off to Copenhagen, Denmark, to present it. That was the beginning of numerous presentations. The first was especially exciting because I was still just a student, and already involved in something that was so important to me.

Still, there were short trips to the hospital that necessitated calling patients to reschedule their appointments. But in May 1979, I graduated. This time I marched in the procession, and made it across the stage with ease. My family cheered, although our seven-year-old daughter, Karen, said that she loved it when they called my name, but found the rest rather boring. Boring it was, but there was no way I was going to miss this graduation.

Now I was ready to find a job. I had been doing my internship at a Ford Hospital satellite in Dearborn, Michigan. I was seeing a few patients there and after I graduated I was paid to continue seeing them. I was so excited about my first paycheck that I wanted to frame it. I had never believed that I could hold a job.

Ford required a physical examination before they would hire me full-time. I was honest about my medical history. Shortly afterwards, I was told my physical condition would prevent me from being hired. I was ready to take it to court, but the department-head backed down and said they just weren't hiring at that time.

Meanwhile, Larry was completing his Ph.D. internship at Sinai Hospital. One day, while walking through the halls, he stopped to admire the decor in a psychiatrist's office. They talked for a while. Keith Lepard told him that he was a surgeon, and was now finishing a psychiatric residency. He mentioned he was interested in working with individuals with ostomies. Larry mentioned that his wife was also interested in doing therapy with individuals, dealing with all aspects of IBD. Ironically, Keith had been a surgical resident when I was in the hospital with my first ostomy. I had told him about the ostomy organization and now our paths were crossing again.

A few weeks later, Keith and I arranged to have lunch. We became excited about the possibility of working together. However, we both were looking for employment and left it at that.

At that time, I was putting together my twelve-week group therapy program for individuals with Crohn's and colitis. I had called it "A Bridge to

Therapy." My good friend, Edie Broida, labored over it with me until we had the program perfected.

Then I received a call from Keith Lepard. He had recently interviewed at Medical Center Psychiatric Associates in the Detroit Medical Center. He had told them about me and they were interested in my work So with my group program in hand, I went to the interview at MCPA. My idea at the time was to take this program to all the hospitals, but the psychiatrists there thought it would make more sense to work from one central place. I left the office and went home. I told Larry, "I think I have a job, but I'm not sure." Yes, I did have a job. I never thought that I would be able to work, and now I had an office of my own and my name on the door and I would be paid for what I enjoyed doing!

The day they put my name on the door, I beamed. I was finally a "career woman." As I was about to go in to see a client, the chief psychiatrist, Dr. Robert Niccolini, asked if I was having problems at home. I was not sure what he was talking about, but I had to go into session. As soon as I finished, I asked what he meant. He said, "You know, we use the telephone lines for emergency calls, and we can't have your children tying up the phones." I still wasn't sure what was going on, so I called home.

Karen, who was eight years old at the time, answered the phone. "Did you call the office?" I asked. She said that she had, but she was upset because, "the lady was playing games" with her and wouldn't let her talk to me. Karen had been connected to the taped message, and wasn't aware that it was not a real person. I asked her what she did then.

"Oh," said Karen, "since she was playing a game, Bob and I decided to play a game."

"What game did you play?" I asked nervously.

"Oh, we just sang her a song."

"And what song was that?" I asked with growing apprehension.

"Oh, just something we learned on the playground. Ta-rah-rah boom te-yay; how did you get that way?" She then continued the long detailed embarrassing song.

"You are never to call the office again, unless it is an emergency!" I admonished her. This was not a great beginning to my becoming a career woman.

From that point on, however, my career moved swiftly ahead. I presented my work frequently and fulfilled the requirements for becoming a marriage counselor, a fellow and diplomate of the American Board of Medical Psychotherapists, and a full member of both the American Group Psychotherapy Association and the American Marriage and Family Association. Larry and I were asked to be on staff at Hutzel Hospital in Detroit, and we started the Center for Coping with Chronic Illness.

At the Crohn's, Colitis Foundation of America, Michigan Chapter, I had become the psychological liaison. In that capacity I originated the "Coping Conference."

Many individuals have benefitted from attending these conferences, which are now duplicated around the country. Serving on the board for the CCFA also led to my writing the "Ask Audrey" column.

Until 1984, my health remained fairly stable. I was accustomed to the limitations of the illness and had found ways of getting around them. However, in 1984, my internist, Dr. Sheldon Kantor became disturbed that my ileum was starting to close at the point of the anastomosis (where they had resectioned my intestine). He felt he had done what he could and suggested that I consult the Cleveland Clinic.

So in 1984, in the midst of planning to move both my office and home, my son's confirmation, my daughter's Bat Mitzvah, the banquet for our class reunion and a shower for my sister-in-law, I went to Cleveland for my second ileostomy.

In many ways it was easier than the first. For one thing, appliances had improved, and the health care providers were more knowledgeable. But it was still difficult being away from my support system. I was very touched by the friends and family who drove to Cleveland to be with me. The doctors again found kidney stones and wanted to operate. They were also afraid that I didn't have enough bowel left to receive adequate nutrition. The doctors wanted me to start total parenteral nutrition (TPN), and take care of the kidney stones as soon as possible. I was anxious to return home, and at that time TPN or another operation seemed overwhelming.

During this difficult period I had been working with Dr. Jason Bodzin on the CCFA board. He had been involved with the coping conferences. He could see that I just didn't look healthy, and he recommended TPN. I was concerned that it would make me an invalid, and we discussed this at length. Finally I agreed to have a port inserted, and we started the process for which I am so grateful today. With the new procedure, I started intravenous feedings six nights a week, but the extra strength I gained made it worthwhile. It seemed complicated at first, but Larry and I shared the responsibilities and soon it just became routine.

The kidney stones were later dissolved by lithotripsy, another new procedure. Twice, I was admitted to the hospital for lithotripsy, but this required just a few days, not like the many weeks of recuperating from surgery in the past.

During the next few years, in spite of the extreme care that Larry and I took, I had a few TPN port infections and required hospitalization. Being in the hospital those times was especially frustrating when there was so much to do. One time I received permission to leave the hospital for a few hours, so that I could go back to the office to conduct my group-therapy sessions.

I was feeling very fortunate to be enjoying good health most of the time. I could do simple activities that I once felt were impossible. I could vividly remember the times I couldn't go anywhere because the car was parked in front of the house instead of on the driveway. Getting to the front of the house at that time, was more than I could handle. I certainly was savoring each day, but I knew that with a chronic illness, I had no guarantees for the future. However, I also realized that nobody else had a guarantee of good health either. They just thought they did.

I decided I wanted to share all I had learned about coping with illness, to make life easier for others facing some of the same challenges. I had been writing a column for CCFA called, "Ask Audrey." I decided to combine the columns with my story, and put it in book form using the same title.

A great deal of my time was now devoted to working on the book. However, it was a labor of love. Years ago, in one of our groups at the Center for Coping with Chronic Illness, a young man with IBD said, "Before I came here, I felt that my illness was taking me for a ride. Now I feel like I'm the driver, and the illness is just a passenger." I was so excited. Through my book I could help people think of their illness as "just a passenger."

AFTER "ASK AUDREY"

Much has happened in my life since completing Ask Audrey in 1992. I remember one day in particular: October 28, 1993. It was a day of mixed feelings. On one hand, I was happy the book was now a reality, and I had entered a whole new world called "publishing." I must confess that I had been totally unaware of all that was involved in producing, marketing, and distributing a book. It had proven exciting and challenging, and also time-consuming. On the other hand, I had just returned from the doctor's office with troubling news.

A few days earlier I had found a lump in my breast which the doctor confirmed was not a cyst. Furthermore, because of a persistent staph infection, I was required to take antibiotics, adding an additional hour to my already average twelve hour daily IV regimen. I also faced the possibility of surgery to replace my present port. Now, surgery for this lump loomed as one more possibility. It had already been decided that I would enter the hospital in December to have my gallbladder removed. Well, the silver lining in all of this was that I would have lots of material for my next book!

Actually, I was finding it difficult to return to the computer and get back to writing. There were so many distractions. For one thing, my practice was growing. Larry and I had begun leading couples' groups together. We had also become grandparents. I had dabbled in some acting and we were traveling extensively. There was socializing, speaking, and arranging for the distribution of Ask Audrey. The days were flying by. It had been over a year, and I hadn't written one line of the new book. Besides the writing, there was another hurdle to overcome: sharpening my computer skills. Ask Audrey had taken much longer than it should have, because my computer skills were so limited. I was determined to use the computer more effectively for the new book. Again, taking my own advice, I set my goals. I could complete them, one at a time.

In the middle of November, 1993, I learned that the lumps in my breast were not cancerous. However, I wasn't as lucky with the news about my staph infection. Dr. Bodzin and I had been working as a team trying to do everything we could to fight the infection so the port would not be endangered.

In December, my doctors decided to perform my gallbladder surgery the traditional way. I simply wasn't a candidate for the new laser technique. The first day after surgery, I was really sick because of a reaction to morphine. My daughter, Karen, and Larry took turns staying with me until the worst was over. It was interesting to see the role reversal. Karen was now taking care of me.

Still, life had returned to "as normal as it gets around our house," until my fall at Hutzel in March, 1994. At that time, as before, I thought I would start writing in earnest. As many of us who deal with a chronic illness already know, it takes a lot of time just to get ourselves together each day, to see doctors, take medications, and schedule whatever treatments are required.

In addition to all this, I was trying to work and keep my life as normal as possible. Needless to say, the book had been placed on the back burner.

GETTING DOWN TO BUSINESS

Finally, on Sunday, November 20, 1994, at 10:30 p.m., I sat down at my computer. That weekend I had heard a poem listing all the delaying tactics a writer uses before sitting down to write, and it really struck home. I had been saying, "first, I'll take care of all my work," or "clean the house" or "finish the holiday shopping." But now I was determined to stop stalling and get serious about this book.

I remember it was particularly hard that day, because my energy was at a low point. I knew too well the saying, "rising to the occasion with a chronic illness, means getting out of bed in the morning." I figured if I could just get something on paper, I could edit it later. I wanted to be a writer once more. It was just a matter of keeping at it, so *Meeting the Challenge: Living with Chronic Illness,* could also become a reality.

That Monday, I presented a speech for the Windsor Crohn's Colitis Foundation of Canada. It was the first time I had driven to Windsor by myself, but I managed to find my way. I had left extra time and even allotted time to return home from work to take an afternoon nap.

The meeting room was very warm, and, in the middle of the speech, I could feel myself getting very dizzy. I knew there was no way I was going to make it to the end, standing there. I told the audience that I was feeling weak, and that I would sit down. From my chair, I finished a shortened version. After the speech, people came up to buy *Ask Audrey*. They had to convert their money to U.S. funds, and some needed change. Fortunately, a young woman named Laura offered to help. People were just putting money in a pile on the table and taking out change. I didn't worry about it. I just put all the money in a folder they had given me and started thinking about how

I was going to get home. I went downstairs, and had a fruit drink. I didn't know if I was dehydrated or low in sugar but felt the drink would take care of both. I was very happy that I had a phone in the car. It made me feel more secure in case I needed help. I made only one wrong turn but arrived home safely.

All the books I had brought sold at the meeting. People had come up to me and said that they could really identify with what I was saying. One woman said that she didn't feel her problems were that bad anymore. Someone else commented that a previous speaker just didn't understand where they were coming from. Almost passing out had been a very effective visual aid, but I hoped that I could just stick with my story in the future.

When I consulted Dr. Bodzin, he thought that I had probably been dehydrated. We decided to increase the fluids that I was taking. I was hoping that I could continue to take them all in six days because having the needle out one night a week allowed me to go swimming.

Soon after, I saw Dr. Diokno, my urologist. We could see the stones in my kidneys on the x-rays, but we still agreed not to do anything unless it was absolutely necessary. The pain in my side was bearable, and "if-it's-not-worse,-don't-fix-it" seemed to be the right approach. During my appointment I encouraged Dr. Diokno to finish his own book, and I offered to share the information I had learned about getting a book together and all that it entailed. In other words, I gave him the advice that I needed to follow. Just do fifteen minutes of writing a day, and soon your book will be done. Once started, it gets easier. Well, I knew that I was started again, and slowly but surely, I'd finish.

When people asked me how I was able to get *Ask Audrey* written. I would answer: "with difficulty." I could also add, "one step at a time." With a chronic illness that advice works in most situations.

LIFE IS UNFAIR: *December, 1994*

I began to realize that a great deal of this book was going to be written in the middle of the night. I had cramps in my legs, and couldn't sleep, so I figured I might as well work on the computer.

The cramps, I decided, were probably a result of too much dancing earlier at my friends' daughter, Stephanie Sills' bat mitzvah. They had occurred before on evenings when I had danced, and then began my usual TPN. I had enjoyed myself, so it was a small price I was willing to pay.

What was more disturbing to me, though, was the recent news about my friend Ina Kadish. I had asked Ina and her husband Paul to take me to my friend Norine's surprise birthday party earlier that day. It was a long day with complicated plans. I had purposely stayed home Friday evening to go to bed early, conserving my energy for the busy day ahead. On Saturday morning I packed a little suitcase with spare clothes and my medical supplies. Just in case I had problems with my ostomy, I felt prepared.

What I was not prepared for was the sad news that Ina's cancer test had been positive. Her doctors had given her one year to live without chemotherapy, possibly two, with the treatment. They had mentioned the possibility of a bone marrow transplant, but that was highly experimental with ovarian cancer. That day she was as courageous as ever and seemed to enjoy the party. Paul expressed concern that she had been doing too much, but she told him about my hectic schedule that same day. We both agreed that it was far better to be active and enjoy what we could.

As for me, I was still feeling dizzy frequently, probably from the accident I had experienced at Hutzel Hospital. I also had pains in my side from the kidney stones, and it seemed every bone in my body ached from arthritis. I was now going to the bathroom more than twenty times a day, right through the night. I had to deal with my TPN and my ostomy, but still, I was going to live! Ina wasn't sure she had that option. Again, I was reminded that it is important to remember what we do have.

Three months later, I had another reminder of this, and my heart felt even heavier. I had attended the funeral of Geraldine Regal. She was David Regal's daughter. We knew David through his involvement with the University of Detroit's theater program. Since Karen had attended the University of Detroit, she not only knew David, but was a friend of Geraldine or "Chi-Chi" as they called her. Chi-Chi was only 22 and was killed by a drunken driver as she waited at a traffic light with her safety belt on. Sometimes life doesn't seem fair.

It was now spring, and I hadn't been able to sit down at the computer in a while. I'd had several visits to the emergency room, a week in the hospital, and many professional and pleasure trips, all since December. Trying to look on the bright side, I was hoping that I would at least acquire some new material from my experiences in the hospital and emergency room, but they had become routine. It can get boring talking about the same old aches and pains and repeated hospitalizations. That's one of the problems of a chronic illness; it just goes on and on. I fight not to take pain pills, and I occasionally feel sorry for myself and wish that just one day, I could wake up rested without aches and pains. However, I didn't want to forget what I experienced at Geraldine's funeral.

I realized once more that life is simply uncertain, unpredictable, and often unfair. Ironically, four of the doctors who had been concerned that I wouldn't make it — Drs. Teitelbaum, Collar, Feld, and Kantor — have all died. I will always remember their compassion and care throughout my many illnesses. But, most important, their untimely deaths have made me realize that we must enjoy every moment we can. We can't expect to get through life without some pain.

I vowed to stop putting off writing this book. It was time to put it together, and now, here it is!

Chapter Two

INTRODUCTION TO CHRONIC ILLNESS

WHAT IS A CHRONIC ILLNESS?

Dear Audrey,

I am 13 years old, and my parents told me that I have a chronic disease. I know what a terminal disease is. Does chronic mean the same thing? I'm too frightened and embarrassed to ask my parents or my doctor. Please, just answer me in your column. —W.S.

Dear W.S.,

There are two issues to address in your letter. The first is not being able to talk to your parents or doctor. The second is the meaning of "chronic illness."

As far as talking to your parents or doctor is concerned, it can make matters much easier if they know what your fears or misconceptions are. They certainly can give you the facts you need to understand your illness. In addition, just talking about your fears is often helpful. Since you don't feel comfortable talking with either your parents or your doctor right now, try to find someone you can talk to. It might be a teacher, a counselor, a member of the clergy, or the parent of a friend. Also, don't forget that your local association has literature on every aspect of the illness. There may even be support groups available to you. Most illnesses have national and local organizations* that are extremely helpful.

The meaning and acceptance of "chronic illness" are issues with which individuals with all types of chronic illnesses struggle. We know that a ***terminal illness*** is an illness that results in death. ***Chronic illness***, on the other hand, means it is always there, but the symptoms are not necessarily expected to cause one to die.

Chronic is also different from acute. An acute medical problem can be a broken leg, flu, or anything that has a definite short-term beginning and end. Though a chronic illness is always with you, the symptoms aren't.

* *see Appendix 1*

During some periods you can feel as if nothing is wrong, and, at other times, you can be seriously ill.

Some individuals stay at one stage of the illness all the time, but this is less common. It's like a roller coaster ride. At first, it may seem completely out of control. However, gradually learning more about the illness, while not totally eliminating the difficult stages, makes those times easier to manage. Sometimes preventive steps can be taken to lessen the symptoms.

Many people talk of the "time-bomb" effect; the feeling of not knowing when "it" will strike. But one can be prepared for bombs, and one can be prepared for a recurrence. First, it is important to do everything necessary to postpone the recurrence. We do not know the cause of many illnesses, so we don't know for sure what would prevent them. But we do know factors that may help control some diseases. Talk to your doctor about medication. Make sure that your body is getting the necessary nutrition, rest and exercise so that you are not so vulnerable. Try to reduce stressful situations in your life. We don't believe that stress causes most illnesses, but we do know that stress often makes an existing illness worse.

We haven't yet found a cure for many diseases; they can still recur even with excellent care. Learning to live with the uncertainty requires great skill. Because there is no schedule for a chronic illness, how you feel may vary from week to week, day to day, or even hour to hour. Others may have difficulty understanding the shifts in your health. It makes it much easier if you educate them. There are usually helpful booklets available at your support-group office. You can give your family, friends and teachers informative literature. You may want to bring a friend or family member to a meeting of your organization or simply tell them briefly about the illness.

It is also necessary to plan your time wisely. Utilize periods when the illness is in remission. Prepare for times when you aren't feeling as well. Squirrels gather their nuts for the winter. You can learn from them. This may mean taking care of activities that require more energy when you are able to do so. By the same token, you can have projects planned for when you aren't feeling your best. For example, set aside a compelling book, a comic tape, or some music you wanted to hear. Having what you need near your bed is wise for days when moving around is difficult.

Naturally, being prepared is a highly individual matter. Each of us has different needs. It's important that you know your needs so that you can tend to them during difficult times.

Remember too that you can have a chronic illness and rarely be bothered by it. I sincerely hope that yours will be like that. Since we just don't know when a disease might reappear, it is better to be prepared and then be pleasantly surprised if these preparations prove to be unnecessary. Good luck, and don't hesitate to write if you have any other questions.

ENCOURAGING OTHERS

Dear Audrey,

I read your book *Ask Audrey,* and I found it very helpful. I wanted my daughter who has a chronic disease to read it also. She read a little of it and wouldn't finish it. She said that you were too upbeat, and it discouraged her. I really feel the book would be helpful for her and wondered if you had any ideas of how I can get her to read it? —M.T.

Dear M.T.,

I can understand how frustrating it must be for you. You want to help your daughter, and yet she is refusing to do something that could be very beneficial. First, as I have suggested elsewhere, you can only help yourself. You can't change others. Gather all the information you can, and be patient with your daughter. She will make the changes when she is ready. You could show her this letter, and then what follows is up to her.

Having somebody who is really upbeat when you are experiencing pain, fear and uncertainty with your illness can be very difficult. Sometimes you just want somebody to say, "I know that you are having a difficult time. Is there anything I can do?"

However, it can be quite a problem if you get stuck in that mode. With a chronic illness, it's easy to begin feeling that you are helpless and the situation is hopeless.

Then what happens is that no matter how sick you are, you end up getting sicker. The helpless, hopeless attitude works on the immune system. Instead of healing you, it makes matters worse. Also, when you stay in the "isn't it horrible" state of mind, you start to drive people away. Others are sympathetic for a while, but they soon lose patience. Then you do not even have the support system than can help you cope with the difficult days.

When I say I am positive, I don't suggest suppressing all feelings about having a chronic illness. It is perfectly normal to have many feelings such as anger, depression, fear, and alienation. (See letter on "Feelings.")

It is important to acknowledge these feelings and also to get beyond them to make the most of the situation. (See letter on "Advantages.") Yes, I plead guilty to being an optimist, but it works. I'm not implying that I do not get discouraged, cry, or become really frightened at times. What has kept me going, and I hope this will help you too, is my ability to be positive. Some of the questions I ask myself are, "What can I learn from the situation? What are my challenges? How am I better off than others? What are the positive aspects of my life? How can I make this situation better? What can I do to reward myself for getting through this? How can I change myself? What must I just learn to accept?"

There are many benefits from reacting this way. First of all, my relationships are a great comfort to me. People are more comfortable with positive feelings. Again, I do not mean that you never talk about your problems. It is important that they are not all you talk about. By being more positive, friends and family members enjoy being with you. That's important because good friends and supportive family members are the best medicine you can have.

Another advantage of being positive is that you will begin believing it yourself. In contrast, when everyone talks about how sick you are and you focus on that, you soon convince yourself that you are really sick.

When you get in the habit of thinking of each problem as a challenge, it is surprising how you find solutions that you did not even dream were available. Your mind begins to operate in a problem-solving mode. You become very creative.

The alternative to seeing the positive side is just looking at the negative side. If you continue looking at the problems and ignoring your own strengths, it will not be long until you become depressed. Then you will have to deal with the depression as well as the illness.

I hope your daughter will take a look at this letter and maybe try to incorporate some of these ideas in her life. Some people get discouraged when they read what I have done, and feel it puts too much pressure on them. It is helpful to know that I did not start out like this. It took many years to get where I am today. It is not necessary to master the art of coping. It is important to begin to find some ways that work.

Again, you cannot push your daughter if she is not ready. You can offer to show her this letter or you can leave my book somewhere she can look at it if she wishes. Start working on ways to help yourself cope. That you **can** do!

MORE ABOUT CHRONIC ILLNESS

Dear Audrey,

In the last week alone, I have heard about three people who have a chronic illness. Do you have any idea why there seems to be so many people with chronic illnesses lately? —W.W.

Dear W.W.,

There are several reasons you are hearing more about people with chronic illnesses. One basic reason is that people are living longer so they are more apt to get a chronic illness. This adds to the numbers of people previously afflicted. It is estimated that one out of every four people has a chronic illness. It's not exaggerating to say that there are very few people who don't have a chronic illness or know someone who does.

Another reason you are hearing more about chronic illnesses is that there are now support groups for most illnesses. These groups usually raise funds to find cures, and work to educate their members and the general public about their particular disease. With more information being disseminated, more chronic illnesses are being recognized and diagnosed. People become aware of the symptoms and go to their doctors for verification.

Still another reason there are so many people with chronic illnesses is that we have advanced so much in the treatments. Some diseases that were considered terminal at one time, can now be considered chronic. Other illnesses that have always been chronic, are controlled so well that people live much longer.

Along with the increase of information has come the ability to diagnose many chronic illnesses more quickly. Previously, people might have had a chronic illness and not known exactly what was causing their discomfort.

So, W.W., you can see why we are hearing so much about chronic illness these days. It is something most people will probably have to face in the future either directly or indirectly.

Dear Audrey,

How many people have chronic illnesses? —F. S.

Dear F. S.,

That's a figure that is very hard to tabulate because there are so many diseases. I have identified at least fifty support groups for different illnesses and I'm sure there are more. The support groups themselves weren't always certain about how many people have their particular illness. Not everybody with a particular illness is affiliated with a support group, and some are not even diagnosed. To give you some idea though, there are fifty-eight million people who have some type of cardiovascular disease. Two or three million people have epilepsy, fourteen million have diabetes, one and a quarter to two million have lupus, two million have inflammatory bowel disease, and one and one-half million people have Parkinson's disease. Forty million people have some form of arthritis. The Alliance of Genetic Support Groups works with more than thirty different illnesses, and the American Autoimmune Related Diseases Association covers more than eighty diseases. So you can see that we are talking about large numbers.

Dear Audrey,

How can a book on all the chronic illnesses help me with my particular illness? —B. B.

Dear B. B.,

Because I can't go into all the details of each illness, I have supplied you with a list of many support groups*. With a simple phone call, (most have 800 numbers), a fax or a letter, you can receive information on your particular illness. My goal is to deal with the issues common to all illnesses. Everything I say won't apply directly to you, but much of it will.

* *see Appendix 1*

Reading this book should put you on the road to coping, regardless of your illness. Understanding that many others have concerns similar to your own can, in itself, be comforting.

Dear Audrey,

I don't know if you will answer this because it is rather a personal question. I have seen your name so often connected with chronic illness and wonder why you are so interested in chronic illnesses? —N. V.

Dear N. V.,

I certainly don't mind answering your question. I'm glad to answer any questions if I think the answers will be of value to my readers.

My original interest in chronic illness came from having a chronic illness myself. I was diagnosed with Crohn's disease when I was just seventeen, but even then I wanted to read everything I could about chronic illness. The lack of information was very frustrating.

When I became a medical psychotherapist, I became more aware of the devastation chronic illness can cause. As I have indicated, the number of people affected is astronomical. The cost to business in lost time, and the medical costs, are beyond comprehension. The biggest cost, though, is the reduction in the quality of life for so many people. A chronic illness can play havoc with relationships, and with one's self-esteem.

And now I will get off my soap box. As you can see, I do believe it is very important to take chronic illness seriously. My fondest hope is that by the time you have read this book, you will regard chronic illness as a challenge, not as a disaster.

Chapter Three

PRACTICAL SUGGESTIONS FOR DEALING WITH CHRONIC ILLNESS

FINDING A DOCTOR

Dear Audrey,

How do you choose a doctor? I want a good doctor, but I haven't the slightest idea how to find one I would be happy with. Any suggestions would be greatly appreciated. —H.M.

Dear H.M.,

Choosing a doctor is very much like choosing a spouse. One person is not right for everyone. There are several steps you can take to ensure finding the doctor who is best for you.

First of all, determine what kind of doctor you need. Today, with so many specializations, you might need a variety of doctors such as:

An internist or family practitioner for general health needs. I call my internist my *booking agent*. He gets the reports from all the other doctors and is also helpful in making recommendations about other required specialists.

A specialist who treats your illness. You didn't mention what illness you had, but some of the specialists are: gastroenterologists for inflammatory bowel diseases, rheumatologists for the many forms of arthritis; urologists or nephrologist for kidney or prostate problems; cardiologists for diseases of the heart; hematologists for blood disorders; endocrinologists for conditions of the ductless glands (part of the pancreas, adrenal, pituitary, thyroid, and parathyroid glands, the ovaries and testes). If you are not sure what doctor specializes in your disease, consult your internist or family practitioner.

A surgeon if surgery is considered. Remember there are also surgeons with sub-specialties.

A gynecologist for childbirth or female problems.

An opthamologist for eye conditions.

A dermatologist for skin conditions.

A physiatrist for rehabilitative techniques.

An orthopedist to correct and prevent disorders of bones, joints, ligaments, tendons and muscles.
A radiologist for various x-rays.
A social worker to help you cope more effectively, or to treat mental disorders.
A psychologist to help with coping or in the treatment of mental disorders. A psychologist can also be helpful if psychological testing is necessary.
A psychiatrist for mental disorders or for prescribing medication for emotional complications such as depression or anxiety.

Once you have determined what kind of doctor is required, the next step is finding him or her. Some of the actions you can take are:

- Ask a doctor you trust for recommendations.
- Ask your friends and family.
- Ask people at your particular support group.* There are extremely helpful organizations for most illnesses.
- Call your local medical society.
- Call your local hospital and ask for a referral.

Now arrange for interviews (be willing to pay) or see if you can talk to the doctors or their receptionists for a few minutes on the phone. Prepare a list of questions to ask. Some questions you might consider are:

- What are the doctor's credentials? Are they licensed? Are they board certified in their area of specialization? Where did they train? What is their specialty? How long have they been in practice?

- With what hospitals are they affiliated?

- What are their office hours, and how do they handle times when they are not in the office? What are the credentials of the doctors covering for them?

* *see Appendix 1*

- How can they be reached in an emergency?
- What are their fees?
- What kind of insurance do they accept?
- Do they believe in sharing information with patients and consulting them on decisions, or do they consider all the facts independently and make what they consider to be the best decision? Which style do **you** prefer?
- Do you feel comfortable talking to them? Do you feel you could share personal feelings with them? Do they pay attention to you while you are talking, or do they seem preoccupied?
- How comfortable are they working with your other doctors or making referrals when necessary?
- Is their office staff helpful? Are you able to get your questions answered quickly and contact the doctor when it's important?
- How long do you have to wait for an appointment?
- How long do you have to wait in the doctor's office once you have an appointment? There are always emergencies, but some doctors regularly book many people for the same time whereas some plan on one patient for each designated time.
- How much experience has the doctor had dealing with your particular disease?

You can add other questions that seem appropriate for you. Remember to have your questions in front of you in writing. It might be helpful to use this book. Sometimes you are anxious during office visits, so jot down the answers as the doctor or their staff talk, or use a tape recorder. This may seem like a lot of work and may not be necessary for doctors you won't be seeing frequently. However, doctors such as your internist or specialty-related doctors are going to be with you for your lifetime. You don't want to have to choose someone when you're too sick to think clearly. Having a doctor you can trust and work with is definitely worth this effort.

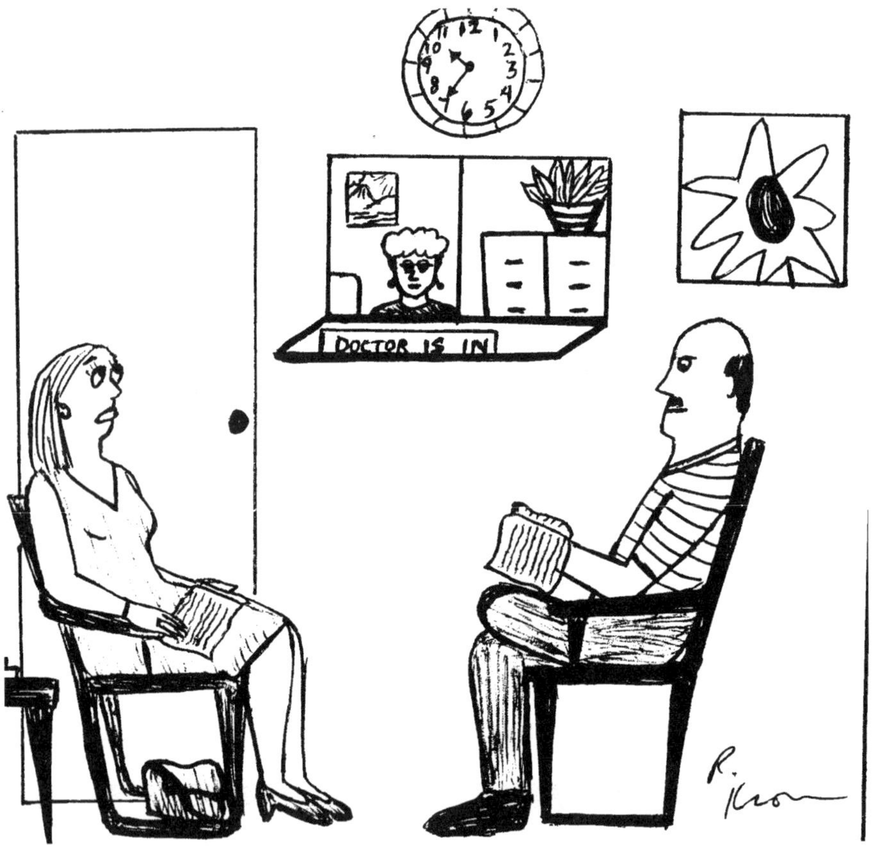

Do you think he's running on Eastern Standard Time?

PREPARING FOR OUTPATIENT PROCEDURES

Dear Audrey,

My doctor says that he plans to do my surgery on an outpatient basis. I thought that I needed to stay in the hospital after surgery. Do you have any information that might help me know what to do, what to bring, etc.? This is all new to me. —L.C.

Dear L.C.,

Today, many procedures and operations that were formerly done in the hospital are handled on an outpatient basis. This may have started for financial reasons, such as insurance companies tightening reimbursement policies, but there are some advantages. We need hospitals when we are very sick, but hospitals can also cause problems.

For example, no matter how careful the staff is, there is always the possibility of transmitting some unwelcome germs. Another problem with hospitalization is the tendency to get "hospitalitis." When you enter the hospital, you start thinking like a "sick person." If you remain there too long, thinking that way becomes routine, and getting back to a normal life is more difficult.

Before you consider any surgery, you should request a second opinion. Once you have decided that surgery is indicated, outpatient treatment in some situations may still be preferable. It is always helpful to be prepared. Here's some information to review before you go in as an outpatient:

You will probably be notified ahead of time to inform you when to be at the hospital. It is usually two hours before the operation because there is much to be done in advance. You might be asked for a medical history at this time. If your history is extensive, you can write it down in advance. If you have a computer, having your medical history ready to run off can be helpful for both you and the medical staff. You will also be told what preparations need to be made. For instance, you usually can't eat or drink for a period of time before surgery. You may also have your own blood drawn ahead of time, so, it can be available in case you need a transfusion.

You will need someone to take you to the hospital, stay there, and take you home. If you live alone, this could seem like a problem. However, if you think about it, there probably is somebody who would be happy to do you a favor. You can reciprocate in some way at another time. If you absolutely cannot find anybody, talk to the hospital social worker.

You don't want to take too much with you. Leave your jewelry and purse or wallet at home. You do need your insurance card and some identification such as your driver's license. Also, bring some change in case you have to make phone calls. It's a good idea to have important telephone numbers with you, including those of your doctors. When you first arrive your doctor will not be there, and you might need some information from his or her office.

Take some easy reading, an article or a magazine, to help you pass some of the waiting time. Check the rules ahead of time. Some doctors allow patients to bring a "walkman" so you might be able to listen to tapes before or even during the surgery. A comb or brush and a small mirror will enable you to look civilized when you leave. Many women also carry lipstick and other makeup to enable them to feel more attractive. A pad of paper and a pen will help you keep track of questions and instructions. The surgical procedure and treatment plans are often confusing, and it's difficult to rely on your memory. It is also important to pack any medications you are taking, so the staff can see them or use them if necessary.

There will be some forms to sign. For example, you have to sign the form that allows the hospital to bill your insurance company to expedite payment. **You do not have to sign any arbitration form**. If you choose not to do so, it has no effect on the surgical procedure. There is also another form called a "Durable Power of Attorney for Health Care," which can be put into your record. That will enable you to appoint an advocate to see that your wishes are carried out if you are unable to do so for yourself for any period of time.

You will be taken to a pre-op room where you will be prepared for surgery. Intravenous lines (IVs) will be started, blood tests taken and the area of your body involved will be prepared. A nurse will be assigned to you and your anesthesiologist will talk to you about the anesthetic that will be used.

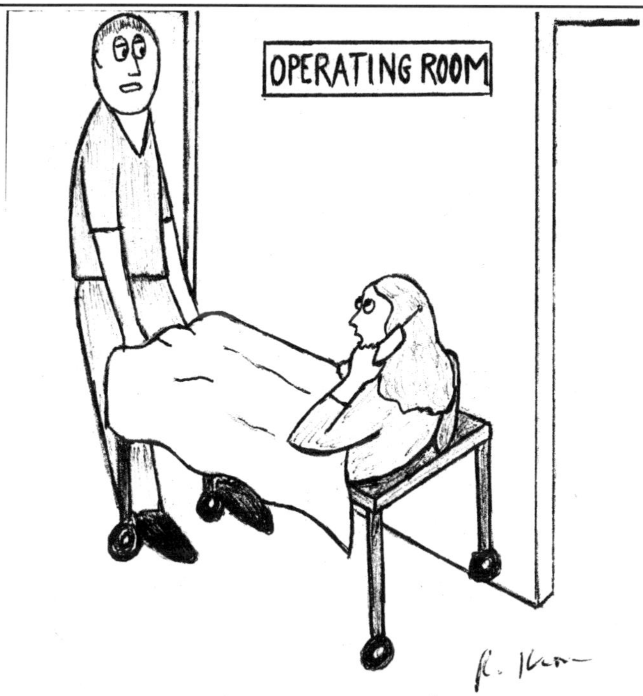

Please, Mrs. Chester, it's too late to get a second opinion!

You will then be wheeled to the operating room. You'll be moved from your cart to the operating room table. You may remember a little of this preliminary time, but before you know it, you will awaken in the recovery room. You will remain there until you're able to be released, usually two to three hours.

Coming home will present new challenges. You will not have the luxury of recuperating in the hospital. At first, you may feel full of energy until the pain medication wears off. Try to make your arrival at home as easy as possible. Just getting there requires a great deal of energy. It's okay to get into bed and order in dinner. When people see you in the hospital, they know that you are restricted in your activities. When you are at home, others won't be as aware of your limitations. It's up to you to set limits. Let everyone know how you feel. Expect to feel very tired. Your surgical procedure will use up much more energy than you may expect.

People who have a positive attitude do much better. Make sure you are going to surgery in the right frame of mind. If you are having difficulty, talk to a friend, your doctor, your clergyman or a therapist. Do whatever you need to do to insure that this will be a positive experience on your road to good health. Good luck!

GOING TO THE HOSPITAL

Dear Audrey,

My doctor says I may have to be hospitalized in the near future. I have never been in the hospital and I am a little apprehensive. Do you have any tips to make my hospital stay easier? —H.V.

Dear H.V.,

I can understand your apprehension. A hospital can be a formidable place for someone unfamiliar with hospital routine. Most of us, during the course of our lives, will have to spend some time in the hospital. The trick is to make your visit as comfortable for yourself as possible. The following tips may help you.

WHAT TO BRING

- Nightclothes, slippers, robe, toiletries, and clothing for the trip home. When selecting nightclothes and robes, remember there may be times when you need to have IVs. It is easier to get in and out of clothes that open all the way down or that you can step into.

Of course, there may be times you will be required to wear the infamous "hospital gown." These gowns are notorious for not quite covering you. The problem is easily solved: for women, bring a long lovely ribbon; for men, a belt. Wrapping either around the waist will help keep the gown closed. Another way to avoid the draft when those hospital gowns are imposed is to ask for two: put one on properly and the other on backward.

- A cardigan sweater makes a nice bed jacket if the room is too cold.

- A tape recorder. This can serve a multitude of purposes. Prerecord your favorite music or comedy album, or borrow "talking books" from your local library (sometimes it is easier to listen than to read.) Your family and friends can also tape messages for you to play when you are alone. Another important use for the tape recorder is having a record of the doctors' instructions. Ask your doctors for permission and then record what they have to say. Often when you see them, it's hard to absorb all the information, so it is helpful if you can replay the discussion or instructions later.

- Scotch tape and some of your favorite pictures of family, friends, pets, or even soothing scenes that delight you. Most hospitals have some provision for patients to hang their get-well cards and photos. You can make your room cheerful and comforting.

- Magazines or books that you are in the middle of reading. It is often difficult to start a new book in the hospital. There are many interruptions in your reading time, and most people find that they need to read one level lower than they usually do. For instance, if you normally read serious literature, you might try a lighter novel.

- Pen and paper. You'll want to jot down questions for the doctors and nurses. You may want to list personal items you want brought from home or information you want to share with your family. It is a good idea to keep records of what's happening, such as symptoms, test results, and the medications you are receiving (when and how you are to get them.) You may also want to keep records of some of the feelings you are having (this can be very therapeutic.)

- Your personal phone book, stamps, and notepaper.

- At least one day's supply of your medicines. It might take that long until your doctor's orders are received. You may also want to show your medications to the attending physician. This will answer some of the residents' questions regarding your medicines.

- Most important: a good attitude. Try to understand the viewpoint of all the people in the hospital with whom you will come in contact. This will help ease the stress for everyone.

IN THE HOSPITAL

Adjust to the hospital schedule. This usually entails setting your watch ahead about two hours, as everything starts much earlier. It is almost impossible to sleep in the busy hours of the morning. You are much better off getting up and ready early. At night, you will be more tired and can go to sleep earlier.

Learn how everything in the room works. There are buttons to call the nurse, to raise and lower your bed, and to put out the light. Ask how they work. Often hospitals have a patient education booklet available. Read it!

Hospital food can be very bland. You may not even be able to have salt. Check with your doctor if you are allowed to have seasonings like Dash, garlic powder, tarragon, basil, dill, etc. If so, bring them with you to season your food. Sometimes this "spice of life" can make the hospital food taste more like home cooking. You will get a daily menu. On this menu you are usually able to write-in simple items that aren't listed (like a tuna sandwich, if you are allowed to eat it). Call the dietitian and write out a food plan that works best for you.

Learn the duties of the various people on the health care team. During the day just some of the people you may encounter are: doctors, nurses, aides, volunteers, students, housekeepers, x-ray technicians and dietitians. It's wise to ask their names and know their roles. For example, don't ask the nurse when you are going home. It is the doctor who makes that final decision. However, if you need to know something about your daily routine, then you'd better ask the nurse. Each one plays a unique and important part in your recovery.

Know the medicines prescribed for you. Also, know how you are to receive these medicines: orally, intravenously, or by injection. Write everything down so you don't forget, as your regime can change from day-to-day.

Know what diagnostic procedures are being done. Ask to have them explained. For some tests, a mild sedative will make the procedure much easier. If you don't ask, you won't know. Take along a magazine or something to hold your interest when you go for the tests. Sometimes you have to wait in the hallway, and a pleasant distraction makes the time pass a little faster.

Be assertive. Unless you ask, you cannot expect to have your needs met. Find out if your hospital has patient representatives or coordinators. They can be very helpful in assisting you with any problems you may have regarding your hospitalization.

Don't hesitate to ask for the professional that meets your needs. Hospitals employ social workers, dietitians, psychologists, and physical therapists, to name a few. Utilize them.

Ask for and get explanations from doctors, nurses, and technicians about procedures you are to undergo. Ask about your records, x-rays, and test results. It is important to have access to them for future reference. Become a partner with the health care professionals on your case.

Hospitalization does not have to be frightening! It is up to you. The key is thoughtful preparation and good communication.

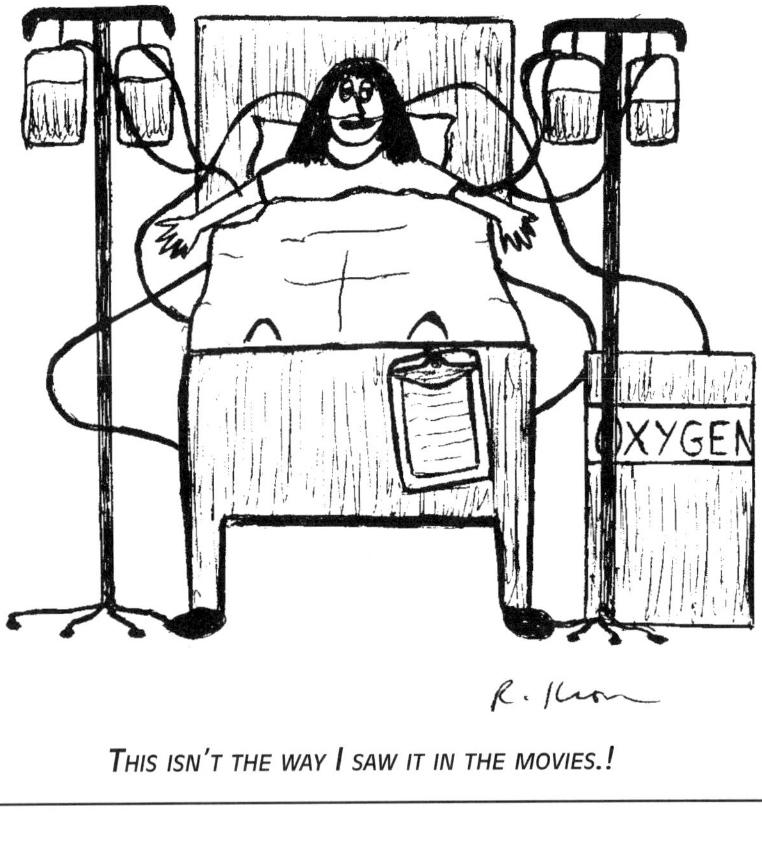

THIS ISN'T THE WAY I SAW IT IN THE MOVIES.!

TAKING MEDICATION

Dear Audrey,

I get frustrated taking so many pills. When I am feeling better I wonder, "Why bother?" When I'm feeling sick, it's a real nuisance. Is there any way to make taking my medication easier? —F.R.

Dear F.R.,

Taking medication is an issue all of us with chronic illness have to face. There are many ramifications.

First, it is important to understand the meaning given to taking pills. Some people feel it makes them dependent, some feel it makes them different from others. Still others may resent the time it takes to purchase, coordinate, remember, and finally, take the pills. Then there are those who look to the pills as a solution to their problems, and they just pop pills with every ache and pain. They don't bother exploring what the pain is telling them.

Medication can be a vital aspect of treatment. There is more and more research to bring us safer and more effective drugs to alleviate many problems. However, we have a responsibility too. Let me share some ideas that may change your attitude.

Yes, we can look at medications as making us dependent, but then, we can also consider that we are dependent on food, clothes, or transportation. We use many resources to enhance our life, and proper use of medication is just one. We don't worry about using water, electricity, telephones, or computers, to cite just a few examples.

As far as feeling different is concerned — that's within our control. We can carry a folding cup, excuse ourselves, go into the bathroom and take our pills. However, if we are open about it, we'll probably find that most other people also take pills, even if they are just vitamins.

Certainly taking medication can be time-consuming. That's why organization is so important. We can keep a list of all our medicines along with the prescribing doctor's name and phone number. We can find a druggist who will mail pills to us. That will help when we need refills. In addition, we can mark our calendar or date book one week before we are scheduled to run out of our regular medications so that we have ample time to contact the doctor to renew the prescriptions. With some medications, it may be necessary to see the doctor before determining what to order. In that case, we may have to allow even more time.

If we are taking several medicines, sometimes it's helpful to take the time at the beginning of the week and sort them into daily packages. Egg cartons, cupcake tins, or plastic bags can be helpful, or anything that will separate pills into compartments. There are even commercial products available for just this purpose. Besides saving time, getting the pills together for each day offers the additional advantage of helping us notice when we've missed a dose.

Another problem that arises with medication, is remembering to take all the pills. I find that a regular time seems to work best, such as first thing in the morning, with meals, or before I go to bed. It all depends on the medication.

It's also very important to know how to take medication. Do we take it with food? Does it require us to drink lots of water? Is it a medication we can take just when we have symptoms, or does it require a regular schedule? Will it make us sleepy or in any way impair our work or driving? Can we drink alcohol while on this medication? Can we stop it abruptly, or do we have to taper off slowly? Do we see the results immediately, or do we need to wait a few weeks to feel any difference? Knowing the answers to these questions will make us intelligent consumers getting the most from our medications. It can also avoid unnecessary problems.

Another way of being an intelligent consumer, rather than feeling like a victim, is to know the names and strengths of the medications we are taking.

This is very important if we should run out of medication away from home, or need to coordinate the medication different doctors are prescribing. We also need to be prepared for unexpected hospital visits. Saying "I take a large pink pill" is not going to help us.

And, most important of all, we must remember our physicians are working with us to see that we get the maximum benefits from the medication we take. It is our responsibility to let them know when we experience any side-effects, or when we have positive results. We also have to let them know what other medications we are taking, regardless if they are over-the-counter or prescribed by other doctors. If we have trouble remembering, we can always use a notebook for that purpose. There is even extra space in this book for notes. It's important to keep a record of which medications were helpful and which medications resulted in unpleasant side-effects.

So, F.R., I hope I've convinced you that medications are important, but it is equally important that we take responsibility for using them properly.

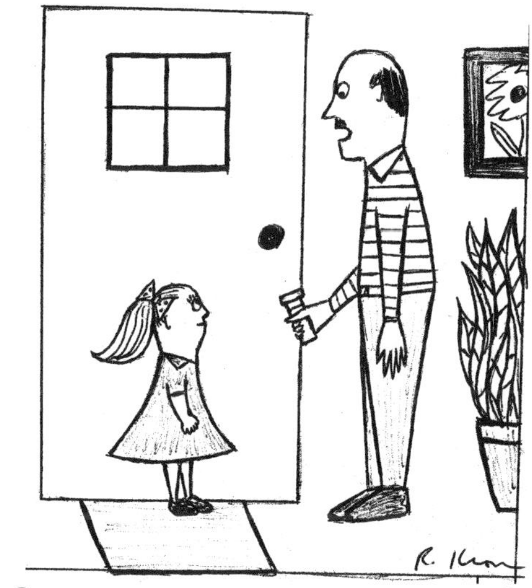

COULD YOU OPEN THIS FOR ME PLEASE?

CONTROLLING PAIN

Dear Audrey,

I feel that I cope quite well with my disease, but I'm still having difficulty dealing with the pain. Any suggestions would be most welcome. —N.B.

Dear N.B.,

Pain is often the body's way of alerting us. We can consider pain our friend, warning us that something needs attention. There are some people who don't experience pain, and this makes life very dangerous because they don't receive important signals.

The first step you can take, once the pain signals you, is to contact your doctor and make sure that immediate attention isn't required.

If the pain is severe, the doctor may consider medication or even surgery, or perhaps just some changes in your activities or diet.

Learn to be able to describe your pain. Is it crampy or sharp? Is it constant or worse after eating or after any activity? Do you also have a fever or diarrhea? What parts of your body hurt? Does the pain shift or stay in the same place? Does anything seem to relieve the pain? It is important to be able to give your doctor as much information as possible.

What I want to address now is how to handle the pain when your doctor has done all that is indicated. It's helpful to remember that the mind has difficulty thinking of more than one item at a time. The pain always feels worse in the middle of the night when that is all you are concentrating on. So one obvious solution is to keep your mind busy. I know this isn't always easy when you are in pain.

When you are feeling well, you might want to prepare some audio or video tapes that will hold your interest when you need to divert your thoughts.

Calling a good friend, or even somebody that needs your help, might work for you. Concentrating on the computer has often helped me get the focus off my pain. In fact, much of my writing is done while I try to divert my mind from pain.

Something else to be aware of is that the body tenses up when there is pain. Then the tension causes more pain. To break this cycle, you might try some relaxation exercises. Again, you should plan ahead to have these exercises on hand. The library and bookstores are filled with books on various forms of relaxation such as transcendental meditation, yoga, and visualization. Find what works for you. Sometimes you can also alleviate pain by just taking a hot bath, or having a loved one give you a massage. Know that most pain is time-limited. Remember that "this too shall pass."

Try to understand the pain. Is it related to your chronic illness or is it something else? Is it telling you something about your emotional life? For example, if the pain occurs every time you visit your mother-in-law, it can help to work out your feelings about this relationship. While most illnesses are not caused by stress; stress does exacerbate many illnesses. If you can figure out what is causing your stress, it may prove helpful.

Your pain could also be telling you something else. Did you over tire yourself, or perhaps eat something that disagreed with you? Keep a journal. It may help you to identify patterns in the pain. If you can pinpoint a pattern in any way, it is easier to overcome.

Sometimes there doesn't seem to be anything that can be done to alleviate pain. In most cases your doctor will allow you to have some medication on hand for such an emergency. You do have to be careful, however, because narcotics may constipate you and cause more trouble if there is a bowel obstruction; and addiction creates its own problems. Keep a record of pain medications that work well for you, and also those that give you difficulty. It will be very helpful to have this information when you need it.

If the pain persists, consider getting a second medical opinion, just to make sure that there isn't anything else that can be done. Another alternative is reading books on coping with pain. One such book is *Free Yourself From Pain*, by Dr. David F. Bresler, Director of the UCLA Pain Control Unit.

During the course of a chronic illness, most people will experience pain from time to time. If you understand it, learn ways to ease it and keep your mind on the positive aspects of your life; it will become bearable. With practice it will become possible to take yourself away from the situation mentally. We have all heard of people who walk on hot coals or endure severe torture. They do it by using the power of their minds.

Finally, it may be possible to learn from pain the pleasure of not having pain. Experiencing pain helps us appreciate the wonders of life during our pain-free days.

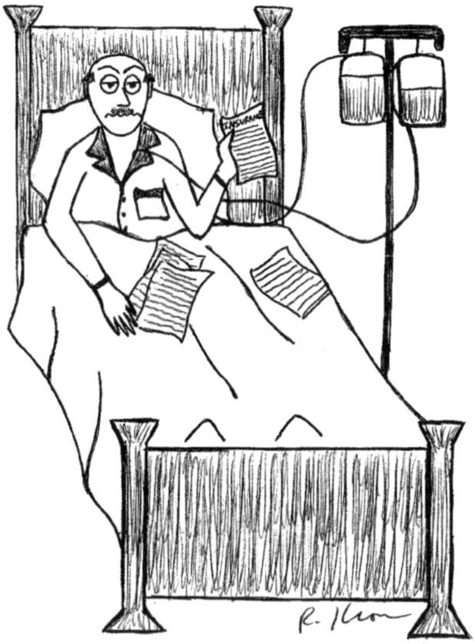

It's not the pain that's bothering me...
The problem is figuring out the insurance forms!

TAKING BLOOD TESTS

Dear Audrey,

I have to have frequent blood tests and IVs to keep my body chemistry at the proper levels. Unfortunately, I have veins that are not easy to find. I'm always frightened when I know that I have to have blood drawn. I worry about it for weeks before it happens. Is there anything you can suggest that might make it easier for me? —B.T.

Dear B.T.,

First of all, let's talk about the agony that you put yourself through prior to having your blood drawn. Often the fears are much worse than the reality. One reason many people fear something is that they feel they don't have any control over the situation. Let me make some suggestions that will help give you a sense of control.

- Get to know the blood and IV technicians by name. They are people, too, and respond better when you are friendly as well as respectful.

- Notice which technicians seem to do better with you. Arrange to have them available to either draw your blood or start your IV. If necessary, talk to your doctor about requesting these particular individuals.

- In most circumstances, after three unsuccessful tries, ask for someone else. After technicians miss three times, they often become nervous and unable to accomplish the task.

- Try warm compresses. Sometimes they will bring veins up when it is difficult to find them.

- Strive for a positive attitude. If you are nervous, it becomes harder to draw your blood or get into your veins. Try visualization to relax yourself. Think about a favorite peaceful spot. Sometimes just visualizing the blood flowing or gushing can create a positive feeling that actually works.

- Do not abuse your veins by taking unnecessary tests. Keep a record of each time you take a blood test. Often, one doctor can get the results from another and spare a precious vein. Sometimes microtests can be run so that less blood is necessary.

- Pay attention to what is happening and ask questions. Where is the best site for you? What kind of needle works best? Are your veins close to the surface? Do your veins collapse? Sometimes explaining what works best can give the person trying to get into your veins helpful clues.

- Don't be intimidated. Be pleasant, but remember it's *your* body, and you have the ultimate responsibility for taking care of it.

- Make sure that you are not dehydrated before taking a blood test. That makes it more difficult. If the test doesn't prohibit it, try to drink some extra water beforehand.

- Give yourself a pep talk. Tell yourself, "I can handle the discomfort. It's for a limited time. It could be worse." Think of someone that has to endure something much more painful.

- Reward yourself. Think of your reward while they are drawing your blood. It doesn't have to be anything big, but just something that would be a treat: going to a special movie, getting a new book, lunching with a friend, allotting some time just for yourself, or just buying something frivolous!

With all of these hints, taking a blood test or getting an IV should be much easier. If, however, you are still having problems, perhaps it would be helpful to talk to someone about it. A professional can help you understand where your fears originate.

You may also have noticed that some of these hints can easily be applied to other unpleasant tests. All in all, you will find it much easier if you find ways to take control of a situation instead of worrying about it.

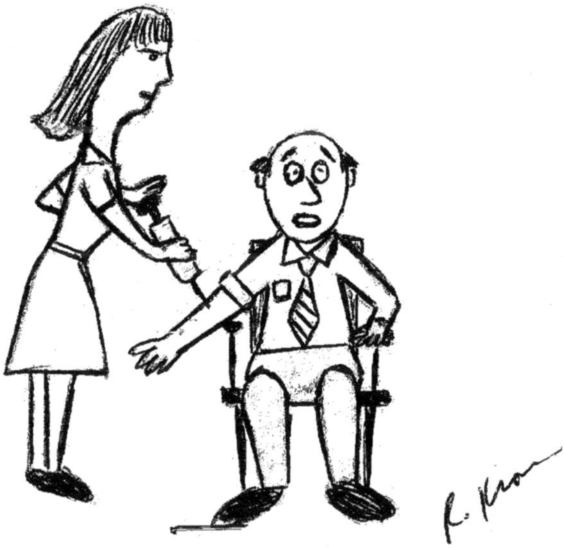

IT'S NOT FAIR...
THEY SHOULD PAY ME FOR THE BLOOD, NOT CHARGE ME!

MANAGING DIARRHEA AND INCONTINENCE

Dear Audrey,
I'm having such difficulty with incontinence that I've become completely housebound. I'm frightened to go any place. How do others manage? —G.R.

Dear G.R.,
Needing a bathroom at a moment's notice can really cause anxiety. It's often tempting to just stay home where you can feel secure. However, my experience has been that most people feel much better when they can get out of the house, and take part in a somewhat normal social life. Some of the hints in the following answer should also be useful for you.

Dear Audrey,
I have constant diarrhea, and I'm afraid to go to most places for fear of having an accident or being embarrassed because I have to go so frequently. Is my illness going to stop my social life? —B.E.

Dear B.E.,
I can appreciate how concerned you are at the moment. Most individuals with diarrhea or incontinence are able to enjoy their social lives once they learn how to handle their situations. Talking about accidents is very difficult. But I have found that once you can talk about this problem, it is easier to solve. I am always amazed by the inventive solutions that others have developed. Here are some suggestions that have proven helpful. Remember that illnesses vary from individual to individual, and also react in different ways for the same individual.

Consult your doctor. There may be some medication that will reduce the diarrhea. Remember that different medications work at different times for the same individual.

Observe your diet and learn which foods cause more diarrhea for you. Foods and drinks usually fall into three categories. First, there are those that are always safe. Second, there are those that sometimes are okay, and occasionally cause trouble. Lastly, there are those that always give you trouble. Stick with the first group for important occasions and do your experimenting at a time when you'll be home.

Plan ahead. Know where lavatories are located before you have to use them.

Learn the obvious places to stop. You can't go far today without a fast food restaurant. McDonald's even puts out lists of their locations. In regular restaurants, walk in with authority and either head for the rest room, or ask where it's located. Nobody knows if you are staying for a meal or not. If you feel uncomfortable about using the rest room and not eating there, just order a cold drink or something to take out.

Map out emergency stops along the paths that you travel. There are probably many rest rooms that are open to the public. Have you tried office buildings, shopping centers, hospitals, large retail stores, gas stations? It's important that you check them out ahead of time. When you are in a hurry, there's no time to negotiate for keys.

Now let's deal with rest rooms that are closed to the public. Supermarkets, small retail stores, banks, etc., all have rest rooms for their employees. Often you will be told that they don't have a rest room, or that you can't use it. Again, it's difficult to negotiate when you are in an emergency situation. However, it is often possible to phone ahead of time to tell the manager that you have a chronic illness, and frequently need to use a bathroom at a moment's notice. You might even give them some literature about your illness. Sometimes that will be enough. However, if they are still reluctant, you can say that you need bathroom privileges to patronize their business. If they still say no, then take your business elsewhere. If they agree, get it in writing. There may be someone else in charge the next time when you hurriedly rush to the rest room!

When traveling, you can use gas stations and rest stops. However, restaurants, motels and hotels are usually much nicer. You can even obtain a catalogue of Holiday Inns along the way to know exactly where they are. If you are leaving the country, make sure you know how to ask, "where is the bathroom?" in the native language.

For entertainment events, arrange for an aisle seat. Ask the usher what time the intermission begins. This will enable you to make a fast exit just before it starts, and avoid the long lines. It's also helpful if you know the layout of the auditorium, so that you are not at the opposite side of the rest rooms. You can usually obtain this information when you are purchasing tickets.

With some teachers or employers, it is helpful to explain ahead of time that there may be times when you have to leave quickly. Remember, the way you tell them is very important. Here, too, some literature about your illness is helpful.

Work on any emotional concerns that you have. Emotions can play a part in increasing diarrhea. Individuals without a chronic illness often experience diarrhea or incontinence when under stress, even though the original cause of the illness may have had nothing to do with stress.

Keep a smile on your face and try not to feel embarrassed. Most of all, remember that you are much more conscious of what is going on than are others. You are doing the best you can in a difficult situation, and you should be proud that you are able to handle it.

IMPROVING DOCTOR/PATIENT RELATIONSHIPS

Dear Audrey,

I am upset with my doctor, and I would like to change doctors. I am afraid that I will not get good treatment if I make a switch. What do you suggest? —M.N.

Dear M.N.,

You didn't indicate why you wanted to change doctors. I have said before that the relationship with a doctor is very much like a relationship with a spouse. At other times I have said that the same person isn't right for everyone. However, it goes beyond that. You wouldn't just leave a spouse because you got upset. First, you would try to work it out. The same applies to a relationship with your doctor. Let's look at some of the issues which can cause conflict with your doctor, and see how they might be handled.

The most common complaints are: that you are kept waiting, either in the waiting room, or the examining room, or that you have difficulty getting an appointment. Often these problems are more a function of the office staff than the doctor. It is important to let the doctor know what is happening. Then you can make some arrangements to rectify the situation. Call ahead to find out if the doctor is running late. Keep in mind that it is often hard to plan what emergencies will appear during the day. If there are times when you are worked in for an emergency, it's important to realize that others may be too. As far as appointments go, do you let the office staff know when it is important to see the doctor immediately? Can you reach him or her when it is necessary? If there are problems in this area, sit down and talk directly to the doctor and make a plan that works for both of you.

You also have some responsibility to make this relationship work. It is important that you come on time for your appointments and not throw off the schedule. Once you make an appointment, you should do everything in your power to get there. If it is totally impossible, then call as soon as you can. You don't want to bother the doctor with every little ache and pain or question at all hours of the day or night. So it's best to write down your questions, and schedule a time to get them all answered. However, if your symptoms are getting worse, then it is important that the doctor be notified. Be able to give the receptionist as much information as possible, so that it can be determined if you need to be seen immediately.

Another problem I hear often is: "My doctor doesn't understand me." As a marriage counselor I also frequently hear, "My husband or wife doesn't understand me." Though there are some differences, in both cases you want to let the other person know that you are feeling misunderstood. You can't go into marriage counseling with your doctor, but you can work on your communication.

Start by scheduling an appointment with your doctor at the end of the day, when there is usually more time. Or ask when would be a good time for the two of you to talk. Let your doctor know what is bothering you. Doctors are often so pressured, they may be unaware they have done something that

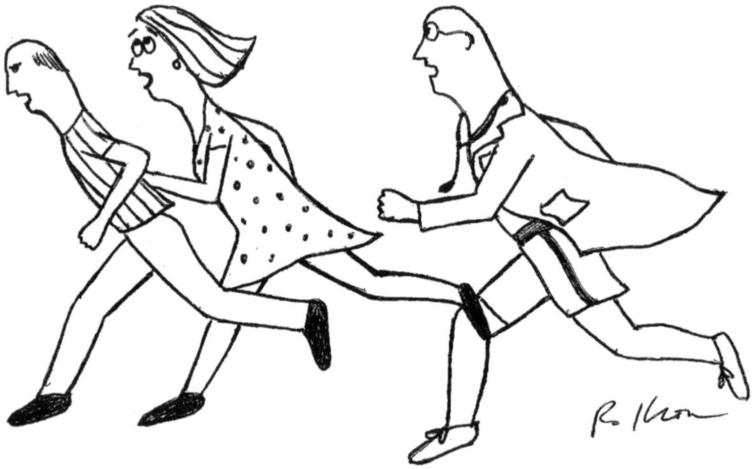

THE DOCTOR IS RUNNING A LITTLE BEHIND.

bothered you. Most doctors, once told, can remedy a situation. Also consider that you might be asking too much from your doctor. Some problems might be better handled by a social worker or psychologist who can devote more time to you. Again, you also have the responsibility of helping the doctor understand you by giving all the relevant information.

Another common complaint is, "My doctor isn't helping me." This is tricky with a chronic illness. Most of us would like the doctor to just give us a pill and make it all go away. However, most of the time, all that can be done is to manage the situation.

It's important that you keep up with what is going on with your illness. Support groups* usually have wonderful literature and suggestions for helpful books. The newsletters from the various chronic illness organizations often keep you up to date on the newest developments. It is better to stay with a doctor who knows your case than to keep running to different doctors looking for a nonexistent cure. However, you do want a doctor who is aware of the newest medications or procedures. It is reasonable to want a doctor who is not threatened by a consultation, or by information you may have found. No doctor can be expected to know everything.

Sometimes, even after you have done everything you can, you still may not feel comfortable with your doctor. Then it is probably time to make a change. It is important to make this change at a time when you are feeling relatively well. It is too difficult when you are sick to deal with both the illness and a doctor whom you feel is not on your team. Look for another doctor. (See the letter: "Finding a Doctor.") Then request that your records be sent to the new doctor. It is important to explain why you have changed. You want the new doctor to know that before you made the decision to change, you had made several attempts to improve the situation. This is an important step because otherwise, you will get the reputation of just being a demanding patient.

* *see Appendix 1*

HAVING MULTIPLE ILLNESSES

Dear Audrey,

I read your book, *Ask Audrey*. I picked it up and could not put it down. I read it all in five and one half hours. Your story was almost identical to mine, except I had my kidney stone in the beginning. That's how mine all started. I now have Crohn's Disease. I'm 26 years old. I am wondering if anyone else who has Crohn's or colitis has experienced arthritis? My doctor says it's common. I don't really know for sure. I never hear anyone else talk about this. I also want to know what to do about it. I have it in both my legs. I find it very painful at times to walk, and at times it seems even more painful not to walk. I'm so confused. Please help! —M.P.

P.S. Your book was very helpful! Thank you for writing it!

Dear M.P.,

It really is confusing to have more than one illness. It doesn't seem fair. However, having one illness is no guarantee that another will not develop. Your doctor is right. It is quite common for people with inflammatory bowel diseases to also have arthritis. Though the cause is unknown, there is growing evidence to indicate both illnesses have something to do with the immune system. **In fact, there are many diseases that are involved with the immune system. These diseases can show up in the same person or the same family.**

We are also learning that the immune system can be affected by emotions. So if we put this information together it becomes even more important to deal with stress. You might want to pay particular attention to the section, "Dealing with Stress."

You mentioned the problem of walking. What to do about exercise is a dilemma that many people with chronic illness experience. At times, it may be difficult to do anything, but then we are told that exercise is good for us.

So we have to learn to both exercise and conserve our energy. To conserve energy, arrange your house so that it is easier to get to the things you use on a regular basis. Although it is important to engage in social activities rather than stay at home all the time, try to find energy-saving ways to do this. If necessary, make arrangements to be dropped off at the door or use a wheelchair.

On the other hand, exercise can also be helpful. Try swimming, biking, walking and low-impact aerobics. You are the best judge on what is possible for you, and how to minimize pain.

Some people find a warm bath helps limber joints. Others find ice applications to be helpful. People often find that the best time to exercise is about a half hour after taking their pain medication, but do not increase your pain medication to exercise. Be aware that some anti-inflammatory medications increase the need for Vitamin C. Discuss vitamin supplements with your doctor.

Get in touch with a support group. There are support groups for most illnesses. I have listed many of them in Appendix 1. Call your particular group for more information.

Many of the methods that you have already learned for coping with your original illness will also work for coping with the new one. You are starting in the right direction by reaching out and asking for information. Good luck. I'm sure you'll do well. Don't hesitate to write if you have any other questions.

GETTING OUT OF BED IN THE MORNING

Dear Audrey,

I have had my disease for 12 years. I know that this may seem like a silly problem, but one of the hardest things for me to do is to get up in the morning. Is there anything I can do that will help? —L.E.

Dear L.E.,

First of all, recognize that your problem is not silly. Many patients with all kinds of chronic illnesses report the same feelings. When we're not feeling well, the simplest tasks seem overwhelming.

I have found that most of us feel better when we get up, wash, and comb our hair. Women feel better if they put their usual makeup on, and men, if they shave. When we're not feeling well, it's easy to say why bother, or who cares? However, how we look often affects how we feel. Looking in

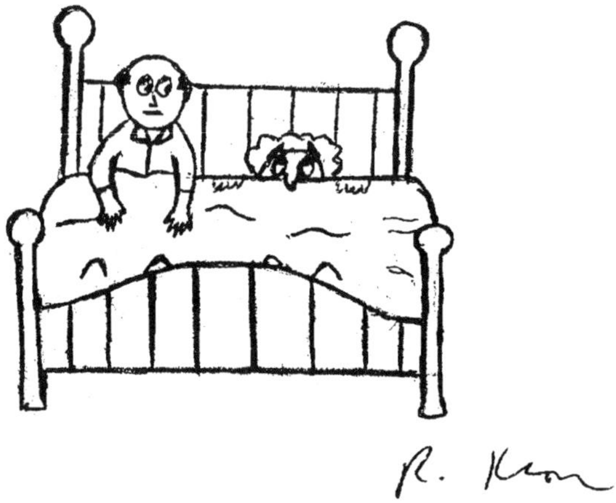

HAS THE WORLD COME TO AN END?
I DON'T WANT TO GET UP UNNECESSARILY.

the mirror at a disheveled person can only make us feel worse. When we look better, others respond to us in a more positive fashion.

Since just getting up can be difficult, we really have to motivate ourselves to take the first step. There are several ways to do this. First, we can have something special to look forward to. It might be something appealing for breakfast, a favorite program we want to watch, a call to a friend. It's not hard to find just one thing that would be rewarding.

Next, we can prepare for the next day as much as possible the night before. Sometimes just little things such as picking out clothes, finding a belt, or looking for keys can make the whole process seem too much to handle if left for morning.

We can have something planned to do each day. At all stages of an illness it is important to have some structure to the day. We need to be realistic about time, allowing plenty of time for any medical care to avoid adding additional stress.

We can set aside some time later in the day for a nap or rest. It can be easier to get going if we know that we can plan on some resting time later on.

If necessary, we can allow a little extra time in bed to just pull ourself together. Having a book at the bedside or listening to the radio or TV can help us get started.

Some people may still have difficulty getting out of bed and may need to consider the possibility of depression. Sometimes sleeping becomes a way of escaping life when it seems too difficult. Depression requires specialized help. Chronic illness is enough to handle without adding depression to it. Nearly everyone with chronic illness suffers from some depression at one time or another. It's no sin to be depressed. But not seeking help is being unfair to oneself as well as to one's family.

HAVING FUN DESPITE WEAKNESS

Dear Audrey,

I can barely manage my daily chores. It makes me angry that I can't do the "fun" things that others do. I hardly do anything extra anymore. I just don't have the energy. I find that I'm afraid to plan ahead for fear that I will not feel well when it's time to go to the party, theater, etc. Is there anything I can do, or must I learn to accept the fact that sports, socializing, travel, or just fun in general are no longer possible with a chronic illness? —G.P.

Dear G.P.,

Your feelings have certainly been shared by many of us living with chronic illness. Although at the beginning it might seem like the pleasures in life aren't possible, you can learn to make adjustments so that you can take part in most activities. Individuals with chronic illness have traveled, participated in sports, attended theaters and concerts, acted in theater groups, taken classes, danced, run, socialized, and enjoyed fulfilling sexual lives. In other letters I have dealt with sexual issues and travel. In this letter I would like to share some tips for bringing additional fun into your life.

The first step is to plan ahead. If you know you have an important evening event, arrange to rest during the day. Allow yourself extra time to get ready, so that if you have to rest or move slowly, you won't get further frustrated at the thought of being late. You can plan on reading, making a call, or just watching a program if you are done early. If you start out under pressure, it makes everything much more difficult.

Next, pack your medicinal supplies and any medical equipment you will need. Once you have them together, they will be available for future outings. Depending on how you are feeling, some of the items you may need are, extra clothes, medications, equipment, special food, and something to drink. A plastic juice bottle can be half filled with water, iced tea or any other noncarbonated drink, and put in the freezer the night before. When you are ready to leave, just fill the rest, and you will have a cold drink with you to avoid dehydration.

Another item that is handy when your energy is limited, is a collapsible camp stool. It can be used for rest breaks. It's amazing how many times you could be sitting and waiting, instead of standing uncomfortably. For some, a wheelchair may make it possible to get around. I have had some clients feel embarrassed using a wheelchair, which is nothing to be ashamed of. In fact, you can be proud that you are willing to do what is necessary to get on with your life.

Another step in planning ahead for some people, is to find out about bathrooms. Call ahead, look at seating arrangements in concert halls, ask others. Even if you are not able to do it ahead of time, allow time to check on the bathrooms as soon as you arrive. Do it before it becomes an emergency. Often there are special lavatory facilities that you can negotiate to use by just explaining the situation. For instance, at the outdoor Meadow Brook concerts in Michigan, a nurse is stationed at a special bathroom, right next to the public bathrooms. By talking to her ahead of time, you can probably avoid the long lines.

Often, the "lack of energy" problem can be handled by just pacing yourself. However, there are times that pacing alone is not enough. Talk to your doctor about getting a handicapped parking permit for your car. If driving seems too much at times, remember that asking for a ride is better than not going at all.

For some people, there may be psychological issues that make going out and socializing difficult. Talking to a psychologist or social worker may be helpful in sorting out the non-medical issues that may be complicating your ability to have fun.

Make these extra efforts to have fun. Once you are doing something you enjoy, you usually feel better. Start gradually. There may be times when you need to stay home. Even then, you can often find pleasurable things to do.

Pick something easy. As you build your confidence, activities which once seemed impossible will become easier.

Learning good time and energy management skills will enable you to start enjoying life. Give the fun activities priority. You will feel better if life is not all work.

So, G.P., don't be afraid to make plans. Learn the various ways you can modify situations to make fun possible. I know it sounds like a lot of work right now, but take one step at a time. I can guarantee the results are worth it.

TRAVELING

Dear Audrey:

I feel very anxious about traveling. I used to love to travel, but now I feel that my traveling days are over. Are others with illness able to travel? If so, how do they manage? I have so many concerns when I even think of taking a trip. —S.S.

Dear S.S.,

The answer to your question is, yes, of course. People with chronic illness travel! They travel all over the country and all over the world. What's important, though, is that, like Boy Scouts, they are prepared. Since you weren't specific about what was concerning you, let me just give some general tips to alleviate anxiety when traveling.

- Have your doctor write a note that tells about your illness, your medications and any treatment that might be necessary in out-of-the-ordinary circumstances.

- Take all your medications with you. Know what medications you are taking, the strength and the frequency, so that you may relate that information to another doctor if necessary. It's wise to carry a written list in your wallet.

- Have your doctor recommend a doctor in the area or areas in which you will be traveling. You probably won't need to use this information, but it will make you feel more confident.

- Learn to budget your energy and not overtire yourself. Allow times to rest. When you are feeling only fair, conserve your energy. Use a portable seat whenever possible. When you feel weaker, consider using a wheelchair for long hauls. Many public places such as museums, zoos, etc., have wheelchairs available. If a wheelchair will enable you to travel with your family, consider it. Isn't it better than giving up your pleasure entirely?

- If you are not yet up to traveling, while resting at home you might want to start planning your next trip away, or perhaps you could take a short day-trip.

- Try to learn at least a few key phrases in the native language if you are going to a foreign country. Try starting with, "Where's the bathroom? Where's the hospital? Where's the pharmacy?"

- Learn more about the place you are going. It can make the trip much more enjoyable. Many books are available in the travel section of your library. Frequently the places you travel to will have a support group for your illness.* Get the names, phone numbers and address ahead of time. Having that information may come in handy in an emergency. Even if you don't have an emergency, it can be interesting to meet someone in a different country or state who is dealing with the same illness.

**see Appendix 1 for your support group.*

When you are flying:

- Call ahead if you are on a special diet. The airlines can usually provide a special meal, or make necessary arrangements if they know ahead of time.

- Remember that wheelchairs are available at airports. Call ahead and you can have one waiting and avoid the long walks to and from the airplane. Also, most airports have chauffeured electric carts available, if need be.

- Make sure you keep at least two to three days' supply of medication in your carry-on bag, just in case your luggage is lost.

- Request permission to board ahead of time if you are not feeling well. That way you will avoid the rush. Most airlines offer this opportunity routinely.

- Look at the layout of the plane and make sure that you request a seat that will be comfortable for you, whether it is one near the bathroom or one with more room. Again, if you call ahead and explain your situation the airlines are usually very helpful and can accommodate special needs.

- Tell the steward or stewardess if you have any concerns or special needs. They can be extremely considerate.

When you are traveling by car:

- Pack a cooler with something to drink to avoid dehydration.

- Take a pillow and blanket for rest between destinations.

- Take a guidebook for Holiday Inns, Best Western Motels, McDonald's or any franchise chain along the way that is apt to have clean bathrooms. You'll have the security of knowing that there's always a place to stop.

- Consider a car phone that could be available for any emergencies.

Above all, a positive attitude and a smile on your face will enhance the trip for you and the people you meet.

BON VOYAGE!

FINDING WORK

Dear Audrey:

I just graduated from high school. I want to be able to work, but with a chronic disease it seems like it would be difficult. I know from your book *Ask Audrey* that you are working. How do you manage to continue to work? Do you have any suggestions that would help me find and keep a job? I really would appreciate any ideas. Thanks. —W.W.

Dear W.W.,

What an opportune time to hear from you! I have just had to take the last week off because of a bout in the hospital, reminding me once more of the uncertainty that comes with chronic illness. You never know when it will strike. For many years I, too, felt that it would be impossible to work.

In severe cases, working may not be an option, and then it becomes necessary to apply for Disability. However, that would not be my recommendation in most situations. Having a job, especially one that you enjoy, can be very good for your health and well-being.

In recent times, finding satisfying work has been difficult, even for those without any health problems. Start by reading some of the many books on choosing a career that are available at libraries or book stores. You can also consult a school counselor. Most school counselors will help you explore career choices. There is usually no charge for this service, even if you aren't attending their school. If for some reason, they can't help you, they can certainly give you suggestions on where you can receive help.

While you are searching for work, consider some factors that would make life easier for balancing a career and a chronic illness. Think about the following options:

- Flexible hours.
- Contractual work that allows you to determine your own pace.
- Becoming your own boss.
- Situations where it is easy to find someone else to fill in for you.
- Increased mobility. If you are going from place to place, you will have time to stop and rest, go to the bathroom, or take care of any other needs.
- Identifying something you love to do. Often, if you're very absorbed in your work, the illness just fades into the background.
- An understanding boss and co-workers.
- Flexibility to design the work, so that you are in a position to carry it out. The disability laws require your employer to adapt the workplace so that you can perform your job.
- Becoming so good at what you do that you will be in demand, despite the interference of your illness.

I, personally have had to consider many of the above strategies and have found them helpful: In addition, I prepare for the unexpected because of the uncertainty of my health. For example, I have all my clients' telephone numbers handy, in case I have to suddenly go to the hospital. Fortunately, I'm able to work with some of my clients on the phone or at home, which makes it easier when I'm not as strong. I have explained, briefly (when appropriate), that I have a chronic illness. Some clients become curious about the TPN apparatus that I sometimes use during sessions. Others are worried that I am going to die when I'm in the hospital. I don't make a guarantee, but I do let clients know the difference between a chronic and a terminal illness. Of course, many of them are dealing with their own chronic illness and are curious as to how I handle recurrences. The most important aspect for me is that I love my work, so it's rare that I'm not able to carry it out one way or another.

So, W.W., look for something within reason that you enjoy, and then look for ways to make it work for you.

MAINTAINING A PROFESSIONAL LIFE

Dear Audrey,

I read your book *Ask Audrey* and learned that you work as a psychotherapist, are the Director of Psychological Services at the Inflammatory Bowel Disease Center, and that you give speeches. I know that you have a chronic illness. How do you do it? Your life seems better than most people's that don't even have an illness. Don't you ever get discouraged? —M.S.

Dear M.S.:

I know that I do manage to make the most of my life but it hasn't always been that way. At one point, in the beginning days of my illness, I thought that I would never be able to work. Going back to school was frightening.

I was most concerned about being able to walk around the campus, and how I was going to be able to park my car close enough. Through the years, I have found many ways to cope.

Do I ever get discouraged? Of course. At times I feel sorry for myself, and wish that one day I wouldn't have to be concerned about what was going on with me physically. When I have a setback I become "impatient" as well as "a" patient. Dietary restrictions are always difficult, because I enjoy eating so much. Medicines that puff me up or change my appearance are also hard to handle. Pain, especially if I don't know what it's from, is very discouraging. Having to plan my life around bathrooms, and at times having difficulties with my ostomy, can also be extremely distressing. And the hardest thing for me that I deal with on a regular basis, is just getting up in the morning.

However, a long time ago I decided that since I had a chronic illness, and there was nothing I could do about it, I would do the best I could with it. In my letter on working, I share some of the ways I make carrying on a professional life easier. Some other ways that have worked for me are as follows:

- Forcing myself to get up in the morning. I usually schedule a patient or appointment which will make me get up and get dressed. In the morning, getting out of bed is the hardest thing I do, and I need some strong motivation.

- I try to pace myself and build in some time for a short nap or just to rest.

- Recently I have started seeing more clients at home, which is much easier than traveling to an office. I also have clients that I schedule for phone time. In that situation, I can even be lying in bed resting as we have our session on the phone.

- I do everything I can to save time and energy. The tips I use in my books have all worked for me. By being organized and not wasting time, I can accomplish a great deal. It is rare that I watch TV. When you think of how much time most people spend watching TV, it gives me quite a bit of extra time.

- There have been times when I have had to stop work because I had to go to the hospital. I plan ahead for that possibility, and am prepared when it happens. During the time I am in the hospital, if I am feeling better, I call my patients just to let them know about when I will be back.

- When I first had my ostomy, I was afraid that I would never give speeches again. I was concerned about being "on stage"—the center of attention. Now, I am more comfortable with it, and I just take precautions before I give my speech.

- I certainly have found that when I enjoy what I am doing, I usually feel better.

- Often when I come home in the evening I am exhausted. If I keep moving, I am fine, but if I sit down, I'm finished.

- I make the most of the times I am feeling well, and have everything organized for the times that I might be sick.

- I appreciate my support system of friends and family, and work hard to maintain it. Even when I am sick, talking on the phone can energize me, as well as strengthening my relationships.

- Sometimes, when I think that I can't do any more, I just tell myself that I can work for fifteen minutes, and then, once I start, I'm motivated to continue. I also reward myself if I finish a difficult job.

As you can see, M.S., the coping methods I have shared in my writings are ones that I have used myself. And yes it is true in spite of the chronic illness I have a very rich life. My body doesn't always do what I want, but my brain is still working and I'm still able to love, and together that helps me have the kind of life I do.

MANAGING TIME

Dear Audrey,

I have a chronic illness. It takes a great deal of time to prepare special diets, acquire my medical supplies, and carry out my medical regime. In addition, I have to see so many different doctors, and take so many tests that I don't seem to have any time for myself. I also am trying to work and take care of our home. It was hard to find time to even write this letter! I desperately need help. —O.C.

Dear O.C.,

It sounds like you have your hands full. I can see how frustrated you must be. Managing a chronic illness takes lots of time indeed. Not only do you have to schedule medical procedures and trips to the doctors or hospitals, but you also lose time when you aren't feeling well. Good time management becomes imperative to keep from feeling completely out of control.

The following are some time management skills that could be helpful:

- Take time to set goals. Consider what is really important. Then prioritize your activities, and do the most important ones first.

- Delegate whatever and whenever you can. Even small children can help out with simple tasks. If you can, consider paying for some services. Even though paying for help can be costly, if you don't take care of yourself, medical and doctor bills can be even more costly.

- Take large jobs and break them down to small, manageable tasks.

- Don't make big productions out of unimportant jobs. We often waste time on projects that don't really require perfection.

- Learn how to say no. It is a very important time saver. You have the right to say no, and you don't even need an excuse. If you do have difficulty in saying no, seek help in becoming more assertive. There are many good books,* tapes and courses available on this subject. You can also review the letter on assertiveness.

- Organize your environment. The initial investment of time is well worth it. Being organized keeps you from wasting time looking for things.

- Use *waiting* time productively. Take projects such as letters or bills along with you. Then, while you are waiting at the doctor's office, the outpatient waiting room, or wherever, you can accomplish small necessary tasks. Or maybe just use the time to enjoy a good book or other reading material.

- Plan ahead. Give yourself extra time, so that you don't have to deal with last-minute deadlines. Set your own deadline, before a job has to be done. Then reward yourself for achieving your goal.

- Gather everything you need to complete a task and then finish it. Much time is wasted starting over. Make an effort to handle each piece of paper only once and do what it requires. Throwing out unnecessary junk can also prove a timesaver.

* *see Appendix 2*

- Have a tape recorder set up next to your bed. This will enable you to learn a language, enjoy self-help programs, hear your favorite music or even listen to a book while you are resting. That way you create a positive experience for time that would just be wasted, and it will help you focus on something other than your discomfort.

- Get away from it all. You'll be able to manage your time much more effectively if you can occasionally escape, even if it's just for a weekend, a day, or a few hours. You need time to "recharge" and to consider what's really important in your life.

- Read books and articles on time management.* Listen to tapes on the subject or talk to others about their timesaving methods. Although this effort takes time initially, it will save you time in the long run.

This is just a start, O.C. In using these techniques, you will find that although your illness may rob you of some of your time, you can control how you use the remaining hours.

HANDLING RECURRENCES

Dear Audrey,

I find it extremely difficult to deal with the recurrences of my illness. I go through periods where I am feeling fine, and I start to get used to it. I make plans, and then, whammy! I'm sick, and I can't do anything. It is so frustrating. I wonder if you have any suggestions. —W.L.

Dear W.L.,

Your dilemma is one shared by many people with any form of chronic illness. The chronicity of the illness lends itself to a time-bomb effect. One never can be absolutely sure what the future will hold. However, stop and think a minute: Can anybody with or without an illness really predict what

* *see Appendix 2*

the future will be? Those without an illness often live under the mistaken assumption that they can, but they are often reminded how quickly everything can change with the advent of a hurricane, tornado, earthquake, war, recession, accident, or death of a loved one. There are a multitude of other traumatic events that can completely change their lives. So actually, those of us with a chronic illness have an advantage. We know that we will face problems in the future, so we have the opportunity to prepare ourselves.

There are many ways to make the difficult days easier. Begin to do so, if you can, during the times you are feeling stronger. At that time you can prepare yourself physically and emotionally for the more difficult days that may be ahead.

If you are prepared, there are fewer difficult days. When you do have a new bout, your sense of control can make it less intense.

We have talked about preparing yourself physically in other letters. Briefly, it's important to set up your life and your home in a way that will make it most convenient for you when you're too sick to do much of anything. It might be preparing a list of numbers of people or services that you can call for additional help. It could be just arranging to have what you need next to your bed, preparing frozen meals, making lists of instructions, having special books or tapes available. Be creative. There are many options.

What I want to do here is deal with the frustration you feel when you have to change your plans. Here, too, you can take some control. You don't have to just give up and retreat from living.

The first strategy is to see if you can go ahead with your plans with some modifications. One of my clients was unable to play golf, because her Crohn's disease was giving her problems. However, she was able to go along in the golf cart and keep score, enjoying the weather and the company of her friends. The letters on "Traveling" and "Having Fun Despite Weakness" both give additional hints. Often, modifications to one's routine, such as being dropped off at the door, using special equipment, or wearing more comfortable clothing, may make it possible for you to complete your plans. Most people report that once they do go out, they feel much better.

Another modification may be in the actual structure of your plans. If you had planned to attend a wedding or a family gathering, it may be possible to just go for a little while, and then leave early. If you are going out to dinner with friends, and it seems too overwhelming, why not just invite them over, and order in something simple? Even if you have to go to the hospital, see if there is some way you can carry on the activity there. I have been able to do this frequently. For example, once I had my literature group come to the hospital, bringing dinner, paper plates, etc. After dinner, during visiting hours, we discussed our book as usual. They enjoyed the adventure as much as I did.

Then, of course, there are times when you're feeling so sick that a total change of plans may be necessary. At these times look for something special you can do to somewhat compensate for the disappointment. What other pleasures can you engage in?

Consider perhaps looking at pictures of times you were enjoying yourself, or plan for some future activity or vacation to take your mind off the loss. Now, with television, videos and computers, your mind can have an adventure even if your body can't come along. You can still connect with people by phone and/or computer, even if you can't see them in person. Taking stock of what you do have can also be comforting. We sometimes are so concerned about loss, that we forget treasures right in front of our eyes.

I realize that just as it's frustrating to change plans for social activities, it's also upsetting to be unable to work. However, some of the same strategies can apply. First, look for ways to modify your work situation. The new disability laws require your employer to modify the work environment to enable you to do your job. Next, you might be able to identify different ways of completing your assignment—for example, working at home on a computer, perhaps even working from bed. Recently,

I started providing some therapy sessions by phone so that even if I had a difficult time, I could still continue working with clients.

I hope these suggestions start you thinking about what you personally can do to lessen frustration. I don't want to minimize the distress a setback can cause. It's natural to feel the loss, and to be disappointed. However, if you dwell on "poor me," you probably will feel even worse. Finding something you can do — anything at all — will give you a sense of accomplishment that will inevitably help in your recovery. Remember, it's not what happens to us that is important, but what we ultimately do about it.

Chapter Four

RELATIONSHIPS

FEELING MISUNDERSTOOD

Dear Audrey,

I'm beginning to think that nobody understands me. I've been ill for three years now, and I'm really getting frustrated. If I tell my husband how I feel, he just tells me to call the doctor, or take my medicine. My friends are getting tired of hearing about my bouts. Family members are beginning to think that I'm just trying to avoid family functions. It seems that nobody understands me. Do others feel the way I do? If so, how do they handle it? —F.L.

Dear F.L.,

I hear your frustration, and want you to know that you certainly are not alone. There are several aspects of chronic illness that make it especially difficult for others to understand. One is that the illness is often not visible. A broken arm is much easier for people to understand than a chronic illness.

With a broken arm, the course of the healing process is predictable. There is a definite beginning, healing process and ending point. However with a chronic illness, often it's difficult to determine the beginning, the healing process is not consistent, and there is no definite end. Each day or hour can be different.

Another factor is the chronicity of the illness. If a person is in an accident, everybody rallies around until the emergency is over. In our society, people are good at responding to emergencies. Unfortunately, after awhile they lose interest. So a chronic illness frustrates others as well as the individual who has it.

Considering all the above, it is not surprising that you recognize a lack of understanding. Fortunately, there are some steps you can take to get some of the understanding that is so necessary.

Start with your husband. Men have been raised to be action-oriented. Your husband is probably feeling frustrated because he feels helpless and wants to find solutions. His way of handling your problems is to suggest something you can do. Communicate with him. Let him know that when you are talking about not feeling well, you are not asking him to do anything. Explain that you just want him to listen and understand. While you're at it, also listen to what he is feeling. Communication skills are so important for good relationships, but usually they are not taught in school. If you feel you need help, there are books,* tapes, and even classes on the subject of improving communication.

Seek out the support groups for your illness. They enable you to talk with others who have gone through similar experiences. I have listed the national organizations for many diseases in the first Appendix . Call the one that applies to you, and they will try to put you in touch with a local support group chapter.

Teach those who don't understand about your illness. Those individuals who are important to you often need education. You can tell them about the illness yourself, or you can give them educational materials usually available through your doctor or at your support group's office. Those who are closest to you could be invited to attend a meeting. This will enable them to have a better understanding of the illness and also open the doors to better communication.

Look for understanding from the general public, although this is still difficult. "How are you?" does not require a dissertation on your aches, pains and hospital visits. Unfortunately, if you report every symptom that occurs, you will soon get the reputation of being a hypochondriac. That doesn't mean that you shouldn't find someone to talk to. It can be a family member or friend, someone from your support group, a clergyman, doctor or other professional person — anybody who truly wants to understand.

Work on becoming a more understanding person yourself. Develop your listening skills. Understanding people attract other understanding people.

** see Appendix 2*

Individuals who feel understood by you are more willing to reciprocate.

So, F.L., my conclusion is, don't give up. Like so many other problems we have to deal with, finding understanding is difficult. It does require effort. But, the results will be worth it.

DEALING WITH CHRONICALLY ILL CHILDREN

Dear Audrey,

I have a child with a chronic illness, and I'm so frustrated. I don't know where to turn. Is there anything that I can do? I feel so helpless. —C.M.

Dear C.M.,

I've received a growing number of requests for counseling from parents of children with chronic illnesses. Many initially seek help for their child, but then realize that the illness affects the entire family. Often the family members' needs are neglected. (See letter on "Family Reactions.*") Some of the various approaches a parent can use to cope are:

PERCEPTUAL: How you view the illness has a lot to do with how well you adjust. If you view it as a disaster, something shameful, or an overwhelming burden that can't be overcome, it will only make matters worse, because you will convey this to the child. If you look at it as a challenge, an opportunity to develop new strengths and a source of greater meaning to life, then you're on your way toward more effective coping.

EDUCATIONAL: An important aspect of coping is to gather all the resources available, and learn all that you can about the illness. The local support group* for your child's illness probably has informative material as well as educational programs that can help you in this area.

* *see Appendix 1*

EMOTIONAL: Be aware that you, too, have feelings about the illness: sadness, anger, fear, resentment— many of the same feelings that your child may experience. Get in touch with these feelings. Try to understand them, but most of all, don't displace feelings that belong to you on to your child. You aren't responsible for your child's illness, and you shouldn't expect your child to be responsible for your frustration, or other disturbing feelings.

SOCIAL: Too often, the extra demands on your time start to limit your social life. At this time, it is even more important to have social support from friends. Do let them know how they can help. They too are probably feeling helpless, and would like to show their concern in some concrete way. Let them be involved. It may be just running an errand or bringing over a dinner, but this will help them, as well as you.

RECREATIONAL: Parents of children with a chronic illness can easily neglect their own needs because of the extra burdens placed on them. It is very important to take time out and have some fun. Reward yourself! Do something just for you, whether it's reading a book, relaxing in a bubble bath, or taking a swim. (Note that exercise is a helpful way of handling stress for everyone.)

FINANCIAL: Turn to the resources in the community if the financial burden is more than you can handle. A social worker can help you find sources of help. Most community agencies have social workers available. Many work on a sliding-fee scale. Make sure you look into insurance for your child for now and the future, and don't overlook scholarship possibilities for schooling. Some low-income families even qualify for free medication. Write the drug companies for more information.

PHILOSOPHICAL: People who have a purpose in life cope best. Some people find this in religion, others in a cause. Working for a cure for a child's illness has been an excellent way that many parents have used to cope, (as well as getting the side benefits of support from others who are facing similar difficulties). Which goal or purpose you choose is an individual matter. Having one is the important factor.

FAMILIAL: Roles in the family may change as needs change. New responsibilities may emerge. Siblings without the disease also need attention. Any problem that the family experienced before the illness is further accentuated by the stress of the illness. Flexibility, communication, cooperation, and caring are all important goals in meeting these unique challenges.

Having a child or any other family member with a chronic illness can be very difficult and complicates life in many ways. Read everything you can about it. For starters, consult books like *Home Care for the Chronically Ill or Disabled Child, by Monica Mies.** Then, the best we can do is to accept the situation, maintain hope, develop a sense of humor, and grow from the experience of a new challenge. This attitude can serve as an example to our children, so that instead of looking at illness as a disaster and giving up, they too can turn it into a growth experience and develop skills that will be useful all their lives.

RELATING TO A SPOUSE WITH A CHRONIC ILLNESS

Dear Audrey,

My husband is having a great deal of difficulty with his illness. I think that he could use some help from a psychologist, but he gets angry when I even bring up the subject. I don't understand. He goes to the doctor when his body hurts, and he goes to the dentist when his teeth hurt. Now he's hurting emotionally, but just the suggestion that he seek help infuriates him. —E.W.

Dear E.W.,

I hear this story frequently from spouses, parents and even children who are concerned about their loved ones, and frustrated by their unwillingness to seek help. Let's try to understand their reluctance. In the 1950s, many

* *see Appendix 2*

illnesses were labeled "psychosomatic." It was postulated that specific personality patterns related to certain illnesses. Today, those who study the subject rarely believe diseases are caused just by "nerves" or specific personality traits. However, those who have not kept up with the latest research continue to believe that many diseases are caused solely by psychological factors. And understandably, not wanting to have a disease that is "just psychological," many patients react by completely denying their feelings. But this denial ignores the role of stress in all illnesses—namely, that illness itself can cause stress! Most illnesses can also be exacerbated by stress. Though therapy can be helpful to address this, it is understandable that patients often feel a need to deny that emotions might be involved. The idea of psychotherapy can also be scary. There is a fear of the unknown, and as bad as things may be, there is also a fear of change.

Those with a chronic disease have additional concerns. Just having an illness is a narcissistic blow. They feel vulnerable and somewhat diminished compared to how they felt previously. If they believe that seeing a psychologist means admitting they are emotionally disturbed, it is no wonder they find it difficult to do. They are trying to do everything they can to preserve their integrity and self-esteem. Unfortunately, they often view seeing a psychologist as a blow to their self-esteem — as a sign of weakness rather than a sign of strength and a means to better cope with their illness.

I hope I have given you some idea of the reasons your husband may not seek help, even when it might be needed. You may understand what worries him, but still feel frustrated. You might consider seeking therapy for yourself to deal with your own feelings. This will serve two purposes. The direct benefit is that you will be working on your present feelings. A side benefit will be that, by obtaining therapy for yourself, you will take some of the stigma and fear out of therapy for your spouse. Eventually, this may make it easier for him to seek help as well.

Dear Audrey,

Before I got sick, my husband and I got along fine. Now we are constantly fighting and he seems so angry. It's hard enough for me to deal with the illness, and he makes it even worse. —C.S.

Dear C.S.,

Often couples faced with a chronic illness will experience some marital disharmony if they are not aware of some of the problems that can occur. Peter Martin* lists several values inherent in a healthy marriage. These include:

- *The capacity of each individual to stand alone, to be independent.*
- *The capacity of being supportive of the mate and accepting support from the mate in time of need.*
- *The capacity for emotional intimacy, physical intimacy and adequate sexual intercourse.*

Let's look at how illness interacts with them:

When we are sick, there are times that it is difficult to be independent. Physically we may be too weak to do things on our own. However, we must remember that even at these times there is usually nothing wrong with our minds, and it is possible to be more independent by using them. One of the most independent people I ever knew was completely flat on his back and couldn't move at all. However, he used his mental and verbal skills to remain an actively involved family member. His room remained the hub of family activity and he was involved in all important decisions.

When we are feeling terrible, we want others to support us, but we sometimes forget that they, too, have problems and need support. They may be worried about what is going to happen and feel helpless. They may be upset

Martin, MD, Peter A. A Marital Therapy Manual Brunner/Mazel Publishers, New York, N.Y.

about the changes in their lives. Anger may be used to cover up these feelings of fear and helplessness. It becomes extremely important to give our spouses emotional support and try to listen to their feelings.

Often, when we most need it, we find it hard to accept support. Physical illness is a wound to our self-esteem. To make up for it, we think we have to be better than human and do everything ourselves. Some people with chronic illness push themselves excessively. Sometimes we don't accept a spouse's support because we don't like the way they do things. We need to learn that if we're asking someone else to do something for us, it is best to let them do it their way, and not fret about it.

The capacity for emotional intimacy can be hindered by withdrawing or holding back on communication. The patient does not want to get the spouse angry, and the spouse does not want to get the patient upset. Pretty soon they avoid talking about any quarrelsome matters. Since many of our important feelings may evoke conflict, we shut down and do not talk to each other, and emotional intimacy goes out the window.

When we are feeling sick or unattractive, we may not feel like having sexual intercourse. But, we can still give pleasure to our partners. We may even get in the mood ourselves. Regardless, it is important not to stop physical intimacy. Physical intimacy is a lot more than just intercourse. It is touching, holding, cuddling, stroking and all of those good things that make a couple feel closer to each other.

The important aspects are to try to understand where our partner is coming from, learn to communicate, and then look to see what we can accomplish.

We can't make other people change, but we can change. When we do, they often change in response. Something else to remember is that problems surface with the stress of illness that might have always been there, but are now accentuated. In that event, we should consider obtaining professional help so these issues will not be a continuous interference with our life.

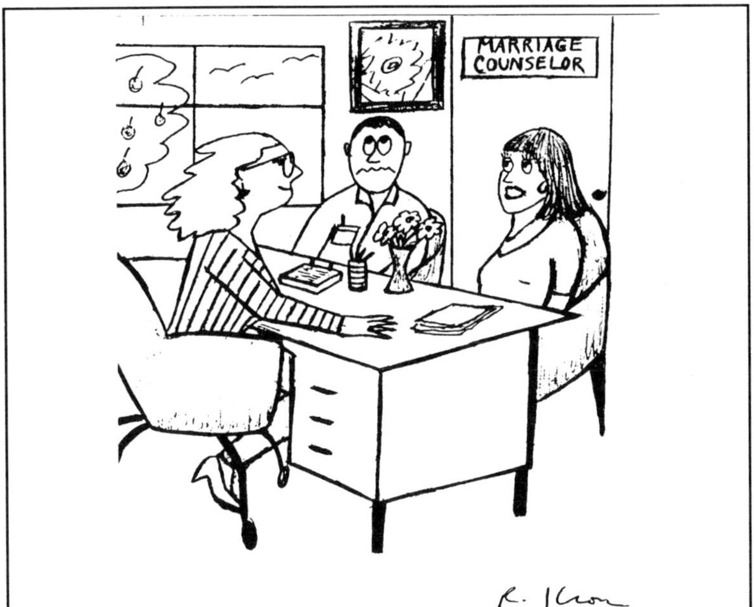

I'M OKAY, BUT CAN YOU FIX HIM?

Dear Audrey,

My wife and I are always fighting, and it seems every time we have a fight, I get upset and then get sick. I don't know if you can help me, but suggestions would be appreciated. —N.R.

Dear N.R.,

Congratulations. You have already taken two steps toward solving the problem. First, you have identified a connection between becoming upset and getting sick. We do not know what causes your illness, but more and more evidence is showing that emotional upsets play a part in exacerbating most illnesses.

Second, you have decided to ask for help, and that is often very difficult to do. An illness can put extra stress on a marriage. For example, there are additional demands on both time and money. The uncertainty of the "time-bomb" effect can wreak havoc with a couple's social life. In addition, many spouses stop communicating because they are afraid to upset their partner and make matters worse. These stresses can affect a couple's sexual life. (See letter on "Exploring Sexual Matters.")

The above concerns are chronic-illness associated. However, remember that every married couple has normal problems dealing with in-laws, household duties, raising children, finances, etc. The following hints may help ease some of the tensions around your house:

- **Tell your wife what you are feeling instead of accusing her**, if something she does upsets you. "I was worried when you were late," will open up conversation. "You never get anywhere on time!" will just lead to an argument. Also remember it is the spouse's **action** that you are upset with, not the person.

- **Try to understand what your wife is feeling.** What's bothering her? Have you touched upon an issue that's sensitive to her?

- **See if you can figure out what the fight is really about**. Are you both just tired? Is there some issue that you haven't talked about that is the real culprit causing dissension?

- **Don't try to avoid fights at all cost**. Instead, learn how to fight fairly. Don't call each other names. Stick to the issue and work on a resolution. If it's not an important issue to you, let it go, compromise, negotiate, or finally, you can just agree to disagree.

- **Give yourself a cooling-off time** if either one of you is so upset you can't control your emotions. However, do make sure that you designate a time to resolve the issue.

- **Read some books on relationships**. The library is full of them. One book to start with is: *Men are From Mars, Women are from Venus,* by John Gray. (References to this book and others are listed in Appendix 2 at the end of this book.)

- **Talk to a member of the clergy or to a marriage counselor.** Somebody less emotionally involved can add a fresh view to the situation.

Remember; all couples have fights. The fight itself is not the problem, unless, of course, there is physical or emotional abuse. The problem arises when you avoid the issues rather than work them out.

FEARING NOT FINDING A SPOUSE

Dear Audrey,

I'm 23 years old and have a chronic illness. I'm feeling very discouraged. I'm afraid nobody will want to marry me with this disease. I'm having a difficult time finding dates, let alone a marriage partner. Do people with chronic illnesses date, get married and have normal family lives? —J.F.

Dear J.F.,

Of course people with chronic illnesses can have normal family lives. However, it is common to hear of single people with a chronic illness, young and old alike, who feel that nobody will want them. I like to look at this issue from two perspectives: that of the individual, and that of the possible mate.

As far as the individual goes, hard questions must be asked: "Would I be a desirable mate without my illness? Do I like myself? What are my strong points? Do I have a good sense of humor? Am I a caring person? Do I listen and speak well? Am I intelligent? Do I have good common sense?"

The list is endless. If we really think about it, we probably already have many strong points that can be enhanced. Sometimes I hear the complaint that someone is too skinny, too fat, too short or too tall, etc. It's more important to do the best we can with what we have. It's always amazing to learn what others find attractive. Sometimes physical features that we consider a liability can actually be an asset. Even the illness itself affects others in diverse ways. One person may find it overwhelming, another, a challenge. What is of prime importance is how we feel about ourselves.

We need not let our weaknesses get us down. We all have weaknesses, but trying to do something about them is an attractive quality to many people. For instance, is the illness the only thing we have to talk about? It is important to be an interesting person. Sometimes I hear, "That's fine for people that feel better, but I am sick and in bed a lot." That is still no excuse for becoming dull. Our body may be sick, but illness does not stop us from thinking.

These days, through radio, television, and electronic media, news and special events are brought directly to us. Certainly we can expand our horizons by reading. If reading is difficult, libraries now offer books on tape. The phone and computer can be used as another connection to the outside world. (See letter on "Thinking Independently.")

However, most of us ***can*** get out, and it is important to pursue activities in which we are interested. It can be theater, arts, sports, politics, photography, cooking, religious activities, travel, organizations, literature or even card games. Whatever our interests, there are usually classes or clubs where people with similar interests enjoy themselves, while increasing the opportunities for meeting people.

Obviously, there are many ways to improve ourselves. There are many books* and tapes available that can help us overcome some problem areas. Sometimes it takes professional help to enable us to look at things in a different way. Whatever the way, we have to remember that we take medicine

**see Appendix 2*

to make our bodies stronger, and we have to pay some attention to our social and personal needs as well.

Now, suppose we are doing everything we can to make ourselves desirable partners, and are taking part in activities to meet people, but we still run into disappointment? Perhaps we find someone who will not accept our illness. Unfortunately, there are people who want perfection in their partners. We should feel lucky to find that out ahead of time. These same people are the ones who would leave when any sickness came up. Sooner or later, everyone has to deal with illness of some kind. These are the people who would not be able to face any of the normal kinds of problems that occur during a marriage. They probably would have a hard time dealing with a mate who became less attractive or even coping with the inevitable aging process. How lucky we are to have a screening device to save us the misery of getting involved with them in the first place.

On the other hand, the partner who accepts us with our illness is someone who loves us in spite of it. We know that this is someone who cares about us as a person, and we have a much better chance of making the marriage work.

So, J.F., stop worrying about finding someone. Find yourself. Make yourself strong. Someone who can fully appreciate your strengths will find you.

FINDING A SPOUSE

Dear Audrey,

I'm writing because it upsets me to see letters like the one J.F. wrote. The letter was written by a young female with chronic illness who said, "Nobody will ever love me because of my disease."

I'm 32 years old and found out about my Crohn's disease eight years ago. Two years ago, I had to have a colostomy. Within a week after surgery I was filing for divorce, not because of my disease or the surgery, but because my husband kept telling me I was worthless and no one else would ever "put up" with my illness.

He had me believing it for years. I spent my marriage trying to "make up" for having my illness, as if it were my choice. Within a few days of my surgery, my husband was complaining about the inconvenience of running to and from the hospital, and how I had to hurry and get back to work because we needed the money for bills. He was on a voluntary layoff for the past five months and my sick pay and his unemployment checks were covering the bills.

I suggested that he didn't have to visit as often and he accused me of having an affair only four days after surgery. I called a lawyer. My husband told me again that no one would ever want me. I said, "I know, but being alone or lonely has got to be better than living in this hell."

With no children, I made it as quick as possible. I got my own apartment and for six months hibernated, crying only to my sister and best friend when I became too lonely. I was afraid of meeting a man. He might ask for a date, then another, and it could lead to intimacy, then he'd find out about me and run. That would hurt even more.

Then, I made a new friend at work, and began going out with her and some other single women. I hated it at first but I kept going because it was killing me to hide in my little apartment, and I knew it. We went to the same place every couple of weeks. I'd sit in the corner all nervous and watch as my new friends got asked to dance and talked to their friends there.

Slowly, I started to make friends and relax. I started going there just to talk to the friends I had made, not to meet men, and pretty soon I had

no problem finding dates. I became a loving and caring person, which also helped me spot the "users and the losers" quicker.

I've met some terrific people, some great guys; a few have been lovers, but none have ever considered my ostomy or disease a problem or handicap, because I don't. The best I can do is help them understand it and show them I can live with it.

I've been the one to break off any relationships, usually because of insecurities they had about themselves. I'm still friends with them. They've all told me that I'm the only person they could really open up to. I care about people and their feelings, and always will, because there are too many people who don't. I could easily just take anyone who would take me, but I found out the hard way that feeling proud to be me is a lot more important than being married just because some guy is willing to. Tell J.F. to go out and make friends first, and if it's God's will, the right guy will come along. If she sets up her own life with a job, goals, plans, and friends to make her happy, chances are, some nice guy will come along to mess up the plans by making her all "starry-eyed" and confused. Life's funny that way. —D.D.

Dear D.D.,

What a joy and inspiration it was to receive your letter. It certainly shows that we don't have to let chronic illness keep us from making the most of our lives. With your permission, I am publishing your letter in full so that others can be encouraged by your experience and courage. Thank you so much for sharing it.

EXPLORING SEXUAL MATTERS

Dear Audrey,

I'm planning on getting married soon, and I'm concerned that my disease might affect my sexual life. Can someone with a chronic illness have a normal sex life? What kinds of sexual problems might I encounter? —B.L.

Dear B.L.,

Congratulations on your upcoming marriage. I'm glad that you asked about the sexual implications of chronic illness. People find this is a difficult area to talk about, and there is often needless misunderstanding because of the lack of communication.

The simple answer to your question is that, usually, chronic illness does not prevent us from having a very satisfactory sex life. But, there are possible problem areas that could cause you or others some concern in the future:

The general symptoms of your illness: pain, fatigue, nausea, dizziness, poor motor control, diarrhea, incontinence, etc., can impede your sex life when you are experiencing them. However, often there are ways to get around these symptoms. First, talk to your doctor. Sometimes relieving symptoms may be as easy as changing medicines. Then, communicate with your spouse or partner and together, find ways to modify your sexual activities to accommodate your illness. You may have to find different positions or different times. It might work out better if you could plan to use the time of the day when you are feeling best. Paul Pearsall in his book *Super Marital Sex** gives this practical advice, "If it hurts, check out why. If it can't be helped, try something else." As a last resort you might check with your doctor to see if you can take a pain pill or other medication that will enable you to participate comfortably in sexual activities.

**see Appendix 2*

With good communication and some advance planning, many problems can be overcome. Some find that sex can divert attention away from the symptoms, but the way you handle these symptoms is also very important. Love, caring, and sexuality can be expressed in many ways besides intercourse. You know how. Sometimes, you just forget.

The psychological impact of the illness. This can include depression, altered sense of identity, body image changes, loss of job, and role changes within the family and society. Certainly sexual relations are strained when you feel depressed or concerned about your body image, your role in the family, or your work. What happens in these areas will have impact in the bedroom. It's important to involve your partner with your concerns because he or she, too, will have feelings about what's going on. Spouses may be concerned that they are going to cause you to be sicker, or that they may harm you in some way. Others feel selfish that they have needs as well. Communication, again, is the key word. How you look, how you speak, how you act, and, most of all, how you care, can contribute to your sexual attractiveness.

The physical changes from the illness. Some fear that they will be unattractive or rejected if they gain weight as a result of medication or experience other bodily changes. These fears may in turn accompany a fear of abandonment. Bodily changes need not interfere with sexual activity. I can't repeat enough that a person who loves you won't be bothered by physical changes. Why would you bother with a person who doesn't love you? Other physical changes may make actual intercourse impossible in some cases. Here, again, is where your imagination can help you to find ways to satisfy your sexual needs. There are many parts of our bodies that can give sexual gratification. If you have questions about this, consider some reading. To get you started, I have suggested some books in Appendix Two at the end of the book under the Relationships section.

The specific fears from chronic illness. Some fear that sexual activity will provoke symptoms, or that one's sex life cannot be resumed. Some fear that sex will make the illness worse. Some fear pregnancy. In all cases, it is important to get the proper information, and to discuss these concerns with your doctor. Also, consult your doctor about any prescribed medications that could affect your sex drive.

With some illnesses, another less serious but more embarrassing problem is the possibility of having a symptom flare up during intercourse. True, this can be embarrassing, but one has to remember that your partner loves you and will be greatly influenced by your reaction. How you handle the situation makes a great deal of difference. You can get hysterical and hate your body and lower your self-image, or you can look at it as unfortunate–but something that happened. Your doctor may be able to prescribe medication or make some suggestions that can make you feel more secure during intimate times.

The specific fears about sex in general. There are all kinds of concerns about sex, with or without illness. These concerns have to be dealt with as they normally would. You have to work on them, or, if you run into an impasse, you should seek professional help.

In all situations, it's important to focus on the potential, not the limitations. Realize that sex is expressed in many ways. Think of the whole person rather than just the genitals. Flexibility, communication, education, understanding, and humor are all important. Above all, you should try to do what you can to improve any difficulties in your sexual relationship. Never abandon the idea that you can do something to enrich this important aspect of your life.

Other questions asked regarding sexuality:

What are the most common concerns about sexuality among newly diagnosed adult patients?

A newly-diagnosed adult patient is faced with the uncertainty of what life will be like physically, socially, and psychologically. What physical changes are going to take place? Will there be limitations? How will it affect his/her social life? Psychologically, there can be many reactions. Some people will become depressed. Some will suffer from low self-esteem or become concerned about their body image.

How do the concerns of single patients differ from those of married people?

A married person wonders if a spouse will still find him or her attractive. Will they be able to have children? How will their sex life be affected by the illness? Single people have the same concerns but are also worried that nobody will want to become involved with them because of their illness.

Are there important differences in the way men and women view the disease's impact on sexuality?

Basically, both are concerned about their partner's reactions. A man may feel less masculine if he's out of work or needs care. However, today the roles of men and women are less rigid, and role reversal is not the problem it once was. There is still some residue of a man's needing to feel "macho" and able to perform, and a woman wondering if she will be attractive enough to be desirable. I prefer to think that these are individual reactions. I do notice a difference in the spouses. Women often seem to adapt to the caretaking role more readily than men do. Women are taught to nurture from an earlier age.

What suggestions would you make to help single patients feel more comfortable about dating and sexual relationships? For instance, how and when do you decide to tell someone about your disease?

When to tell someone about your illness depends on when you sense that the relationship is more than casual. It is not necessarily the first thing you would say. Telling someone you have some health problems may be a start. It is important to explain your illness and how it affects you. Sharing literature or going to a support group meeting with your date can be helpful. The important issue is how you present it. If you seem overwhelmed, others will be too. If you can take the illness in stride, you may find that others can as well. (Also see letter on "Finding a Spouse.")

What advice would you give a couple who hope to have children?

Most couples have no difficulty conceiving. However, medication, surgery, and some illnesses can result in infertility.

In cases of infertility, all avenues should be considered. Infertility specialists now have many new methods available. If conception isn't possible, adoption is also an alternative. Children bond with the parents who raise them. Adoption procedures should be started as soon as possible, since it sometimes takes a very long time. If these steps do not work out, there are still other ways for you to bring love to a child. You might investigate a foster-children's program, participate in big-brother or big-sister organizations, or learn about an individual child or group of children who would benefit from your caring about them.

Some people who are ill may avoid sexual relationships because of self-consciousness about their illness. What advice can you give to such patients?

Sexual relationships are an important aspect of being a whole person. Before you rule out this side of your life, it might be advisable to seek professional guidance. On the lighter side, it helps to remember that most people are self-conscious about sexual relationships. People are always wondering what others think about them. Those who aren't dealing with an illness may be dealing with other difficulties about how they perceive their bodies, such as feeling they are too fat, too thin, too short, too tall, etc.

If a patient is having difficulty coping sexually, at what point should professional help be considered? What does therapy entail?

If you are feeling anger, guilt, resentment, depression or lack of self-esteem and have difficulty dealing with these feelings yourself, therapy could be useful. A simple guideline is to notice if you are feeling unhappy and also feeling helpless about doing anything about it. Then it may be time to talk to a professional.

The first step is getting an evaluation. Sometimes treatment can be limited to sex therapy, where you learn techniques to help you work out sexual problems. Sometimes there are other issues in a relationship. If there were even slight problems before, illness can exacerbate them. In this case, a marriage counselor can be recommended. Most often, when there are problems, they are the result of individual issues which require someone trained in understanding individual dynamics—why we act the way we do. The same therapist might be skilled in all three approaches, but the emphasis is different.

Organizations* can be called upon to recommend credentialed therapists in your area. Hospitals and universities can also be resources, or you can ask friends. Sometimes your local chapter has therapists who are aware of the special needs of chronic illness patients. In all of the above therapies, it is important that the therapist understand the illness and what part it plays in the difficulties. The main purpose of therapy is to help you understand what is preventing you from accomplishing what you desire.

What is the role of a support group in helping patients deal with sexuality and chronic illness?

Support groups** enable a person to know that he or she is not alone. Furthermore, it adds to everyone's self-esteem to be able to help someone else. Support groups aid in obtaining information and in giving encouragement. Just talking about the issues related to chronic illness can often alleviate stress.

** see page 112 for organizations.*
***see Appendix 1*

The following organizations have specific requirements for membership. They can refer therapists who have met these requirements. For more information write or call:

American Association for Marriage and Family Therapy
1133 15th Street NW
Washington, D.C. 20005
(202) 452-0109

American Association of Sex Educators, Counselors, and Therapists
P.O. Box 238
Mount Vernon, Ia.
(319) 895-8407

The National Registry of Certified Group Psychotherapists
25 East 21st Street, 6th floor
New York, New York 10010
(212) 477-1600 fax: (212) 979-6627

BUILDING FRIENDSHIPS

Dear Audrey,

One of the concerns that I have is how to make and keep friends when I have an illness. Sometimes I find it easier just not to see people. —R.K.

Dear R.K.,

Friends are very important, especially if you have a chronic illness. There are many ways to make and maintain friendships, despite the limitations of chronic illness. Let's look at some of them:

- Let your friends help you. They may feel helpless, too. They may want to do something, but not know what to do. Asking them to do a small task can relieve their sense of helplessness. You may need a ride to the doctor, a dinner brought in, or just a phone call or visit. It makes people feel better to be told specifically how they may help you.

- Limit talking about your illness. It's tempting, when something is hurting, to tell everybody all the details. You can get a reputation as a hypochondriac. Others may be interested for a while, but they will become uncomfortable when you elaborate too often. If every time they ask how you feel, you say, "My stomach hurts; I feel terrible, etc.," eventually they'll stop asking. Share your feelings about your illness with some people, but be selective. Make sure they really want to hear.

- Be an interesting person. You cannot blame people for not wanting to be around if your illness is the only topic of conversation. Read the newspaper. Listen to talk shows. Become aware of the world around you. Remember that you are not just an illness; you are a person, with all kinds of ideals, values, and opinions.

- Be a friend. If you want friends, you have to care about others and be considerate of their needs. During times when you are feeling better, it's important to help your friends and be supportive.

- Accept your friends and their flaws. Nobody's perfect. If you look for acceptance, learn to be more accepting. Talk about problem areas in your friendship. Try to identify how the problems make you feel and what can be done to solve them.

- Get involved in organizations. Help others that are less fortunate. You will not only have more interesting causes to talk about, but you might even meet some new people along the way. Your local support organization* is a great place to start.

**see Appendix 1*

- Make an effort to keep social appointments and be prompt. Of course, this can be very difficult with a chronic illness. Allow yourself extra time and plan to rest if necessary.

- Try to adapt situations. Instead of saying, "I can't go," make the situation one you can handle. Again, use your creativity. Sometimes advanced planning may be required, like checking out if the bathroom or the physical area is convenient for you. You may have to make special arrangements for food, or for being dropped off at the door, etc. Do what it takes to make yourself as comfortable as possible.

- Don't be afraid to share your feelings. Making yourself vulnerable allows your friends to do the same and creates closeness.

- Take the initiative with social activities. Don't stand on ceremony waiting for someone to call you. There is someone that would be happy to hear from you right now!

Your medical treatment is very important R.K., but don't underestimate the power and support of your friends. Good friends are treasures that will help you through some of the more difficult times. Work on finding and keeping a circle of friends.

BEING A GOOD VISITOR

Dear Audrey,

My best friend is in the hospital, and I want to support her as much as I can. I don't want to do anything that could be harmful. I would really appreciate it if you would give me any suggestions on how to be as helpful as possible. —W.W.

Dear W.W.,

Just knowing that you want to support her while she is in the hospital will be very comforting to your friend. There are other actions you can take that would also be appreciated.

Call before you go to the hospital. See if your friend is up to receiving company. If you say that you are coming, make sure that you follow through and come when you said you would. People in the hospital may plan their day around your visit, and it can be very disappointing if you don't show up. Also, ask if there is something you can bring your friend. Don't leave it vague like, "Is there anything you need?" Make some specific suggestions such as, "Do you want me to bring you some lunch, or some clothes from home," or "Could you use some new reading material?"

Once you arrive at the hospital, you can consider these suggestions:

- Ask if there is anything your friend would like you to do for her.

- Inquire if she wants you to water the flowers, brush her hair, or straighten the room. It might be helpful to write down the gifts she has received or help her fill out her menu. Often if you don't suggest anything, your friend may hesitate to ask for help.

- Ask about her health and her day. This isn't the time to unload your problems. Be sensitive to her mood and needs.

- Think of a good joke or piece of interesting news you can share with her.

- Do not come with a large group of people. If there are more than two or three people already there, wait until somebody leaves. Large groups can be overwhelming for someone who is trying to deal with an illness.

- Do not stay too long. A half hour is more than enough in most circumstances. If you see that your friend is getting tired, make your visit even shorter.

- Offer to wait outside, if a doctor or nurse comes in while you are there. There are times when your friend may want some privacy.

Another question I am often asked is, "**What can I bring as a present for someone in the hospital?**" Some of the following are usually welcome gifts:

- Stationery, thank-you notes, pen and stamps.
- Books that are easy to read. Humorous books are always good.
- Magazines or interesting articles are also welcome.
- Tape recorders and tapes. They are sometimes easier to handle than reading material. Your friend's favorite music, some comedy tapes, or even messages from her family and friends can all be played when she is too weak to do anything else.
- Flowers, plants, or anything to decorate the room. You don't have to spend a great deal of money on expensive flowers. Sometimes just a few flowers in a bud vase can be replenished at each visit and enjoyed even more.
- Nightgowns, robes, bed jackets, pajamas. These give a welcome change from the hospital gowns. Try to find ones that are easy to get in and out of, and allow IVs to be administered. Something that buttons up is usually a safe bet.
- Cologne, talcum powder, or other toiletries are usually welcome treats.
- Photographs you think your friend would enjoy. These can be put in a small album. They can be reminders of happy days and loving people.
- Fun jewelry or badges to wear on hospital attire. You don't want anything expensive, but a cute pin, badge, or pair of earrings could cheer her up or serve as a conversation piece for people coming into the room.

- Balloons. Many people send balloons these days. They are cheerful, but be aware that some hospitals have rules forbidding them. It is wise to check the hospital's policy first.
- Food. Hospital food is not known for its gourmet features. Check first to see what kind of diet your friend is on. Fancy teas or ices are nice when a liquid diet is required. When all solid food is allowed, check to see what sounds appealing. A novel idea would be to put many different spices such as dill, garlic, basil, Dash etc. in little jars, to spice up the bland food. Something to snack on between meals is usually welcome. Depending on your friend's taste, it can be candy, cookies, or a healthy snack.

There are also ways to help, even when you cannot be at the hospital. Cards are always appreciated and can be looked at over and over again. Adding little notes or a joke makes them even more special.

Calls are also a way to let your friend know you are thinking about her. Always preface the call with, "Is this a good time for you to talk?" If it is not, find out when a good time would be.

Keep your calls short and positive. Again this isn't the time to discuss your problems. When your friend starts to recover, she may want to be more involved in your life. In the early days of hospitalization, it may be difficult for your friend to reach out to someone else.

Let your friend know that you are willing to help. Again, be specific. If you say, "Is there anything I can do?" The answer is usually, "No." Instead ask if you can bring a meal, run an errand, water plants at home, drive a child to an appointment, mail some letters, drive her home from the hospital or make some phone calls.

I hope these suggestions are useful. However, just communicating with your friend that you want to help, is more support than you realize. Knowing that our friends and family are there for us, makes it easier to get through the difficult times. A side benefit is that going through these difficult times together will often bring good friends closer.

Chapter Five

FAMILY MEMBERS' PERSPECTIVES

DEALING WITH DOCTORS
A FAMILY MEMBER'S PERSPECTIVE

by Lawrence Kron, Ph.D.

In order to be as helpful as possible to the patient we, as family members, find ourselves in constant search of information. Whether it's about the disease itself, or how the patient is feeling today, or what is the current prognosis, we are all comforted by learning as much as we can. We feel more comfortable when we eliminate uncertainty. Educating ourselves as much as we can, is a way I recommend being of help to the patient.

However, some problems can arise even when we are, with the best of intentions, trying to help our family member in this way. One problem seems to arise consistently. It occurs when we try to learn more about their situation by contacting their physician. Doing so tends to place the physician in an awkward position because the physician has an ethical obligation to keep the patient's confidence. It is often for this reason that family members say they are uneasy about the patient's physician. Somehow they experience the responses they receive as somewhat vague. They are usually right. The physician is struggling with a desire to tell them as much as possible, while at the same time fulfilling an ethical obligation.

The patient may also object, feeling that a right to privacy has been intruded upon. Well then, are we supposed to ask no questions and suffer in silence? How do we educate ourselves if we can't talk to the doctor? The answer is that we are most respectful of a patient's right to privacy when we acknowledge it. We need only ask the patient, first, if it's all right with them to speak to the doctor. Having the patient's permission honors his/her right to privacy and also releases the physician from any ethical constraints.

Asking the patient before talking to the doctor has another potential benefit. In contrast to the situation we've been discussing, some patients think we don't care about them if we don't want to talk to their physician.

Assuming that we will be invading their privacy may be incorrect. Asking them first merely shows that we respect their needs enough to subordinate our own for the moment. Our willingness to let the patient decide about speaking to his/her doctor is often more valuable to the patient than actually having the information we will obtain.

The most surprising thing for most family members is that, once we have asked for permission, whether we talk to the physician or not usually isn't so important to the patient. It's the asking that counted most! And it's usually the case that permission is granted.

MANAGING TIME FROM A FAMILY MEMBER'S PERSPECTIVE

by Lawrence Kron, Ph.D.

We have talked previously about the seemingly overwhelming demands upon their time that patients experience. Let us now try to look at the same problem from the standpoint of family members.

The need to prioritize tasks and to prepare in advance for changes in plans has been pointed out. It's worth taking a moment to recall that setting priorities helps us to feel the greatest sense of accomplishment possible under the pressure of time. Suppose, for instance, we have spent time during the day looking around the new shopping center that just opened even though we have some work left to do at the office that will be needed the next day. We will be more than a little frustrated if we are suddenly called upon to help out at home because the patient is not feeling well. If we had done the report before taking time off to tour the mall, we would be better able to handle the unexpected situation. In effect, by planning ahead, we would have partly prepared for what happened. Preparing in advance for possible changes in plans helps to take some of the edge of annoyance away from what would otherwise be a very frustrating situation.

While the problems we face are not always quite so simple, there is a general principle that can help us if we keep it in mind: Don't waste time trying to change something that is out of our control. For example, it does little good to give the patient unsolicited advice about how to feel better at the very time the patient is experiencing discomfort. We can't do anything about how the patient feels at the moment. It is much more effective to concentrate on what we can do. We can decide how to spend the extra time available because we had to cancel our plans; for example — do something to lighten the patient's burden, such as bringing medications, or fixing the evening meal, reading a book, or seeing that movie that the patient didn't want to see anyway.

If we accept the idea that living with a chronic illness in the family will create unexpected demands on our time when we aren't always expecting it, we can make some adjustments. One way is to make as many of the menial, or ordinary tasks we do at home as routine as possible. We can try to take out the garbage or do the dishes or pay our bills at the same time each day or week. Having to remember the little things becomes a burden when we're under the added pressure of an exacerbation of the illness. When we make the little things a routine part of our lives, we don't have to give them any extra thought. Then, we may be better able to handle the unexpected extra pressures as they arise.

HANDLING RECURRENCES
A FAMILY MEMBER'S PERSPECTIVE

by Lawrence Kron, Ph.D.

Earlier we dealt with the problem of changing plans because of a recurrence of a chronic illness. We looked at the problem from the patient's point of view. I'd now like to look at the situation from the family member's or significant other's point of view. For sake of convenience, I refer to spouses.

I'll leave it to you to translate the ideas to your specific relationship, parent-child, brother-sister, friend, etc.

It should go without saying that sudden changes do occur in all our lives. Loss of a job, a natural disaster, an automobile accident can dash our hopes in one way or another. We all wish life could be more predictable. That is often the source of our difficulty when illness recurs. We want so badly to have a "normal" life that we come to expect it when things have been going well for us.

The key to living with the disruptions caused by our spouse's recurrence is planning in advance. For instance, if you plan a day at the beach with friends, you are very disappointed if it rains. But if you've planned in advance to go to the beach if the sun is out and to go to a movie if it is cloudy or rains, your sense of disappointment is substantially diminished. The circumstance is the same, but its effect upon you is very different if you've planned ahead. The idea is not to put all of your eggs in one basket.

A flare-up of an illness or even a brief recurrence of symptoms in your spouse can be very frustrating, especially if you are in the process of leaving home to go to a party or an important activity. However, if you expect delays to occur on occasion, and you have on hand a book or magazine that you'd like to read, you feel differently. And you'd be amazed how much useful reading you can complete while you're waiting for your spouse. The best part, however, is that you will be in a better mood and will be better able to enjoy whatever you do choose to do. Of course, there are times when your spouse will need your help. At those times, you can go ahead with what's needed but still be thinking of ways to satisfy some of your needs in the future.

Because the interruption of plans usually comes without warning, it's important that your plans have some flexibility built into them. For example, it's hard to deal with an interruption to plans to go dancing. It's somewhat easier to handle if your plans were to dance if you could, but you'd also be happy just listening to the music being played.

Sometimes your plans aren't just delayed, but they have to be canceled altogether. Again, having options available eases the burden. Just because your spouse is having a problem doesn't mean that you have to be a martyr. Think about it. If you were ill, would you always want your spouse to sit around and mope? Or would you prefer that he/she had some fun and came back and told you about it? You can help your spouse get as comfortable as possible at home and then go out and enjoy the alternative you planned for yourself. If you return home in a good mood, it will reduce any guilt your spouse might feel about "spoiling your plans."

If your activity was couple oriented, your plans might have to be canceled. However, you can still make fall-back arrangements. If you can't go out, perhaps there are other joint activities that you can plan to do together at home. You might want to make yourselves comfortable and watch a movie together, or play cards or a board game. The possibilities are endless. It can even be fun making a list of ideas, so long as you do it in advance. When the situation arises, just pull out the list. Planning ahead makes all the difference.

FAMILY REACTIONS

—Lawrence Kron, Ph.D.

There is no experience which quite equals that which occurs when a member of our family is stricken by an illness. When we are dealing with a chronic illness, the experience is repeated each time there is an exacerbation of the illness. Often ignored in the process, are the stresses and strains undergone by the family members. This section is intended to make us more aware of their needs, which are often inadvertently cast aside. Only by recognizing these needs can we hope to relieve some of the pressures they experience.

One of the first difficulties family members confront is the anxiety engendered by not knowing what is going on with the patient. This problem parallels the patient's own concerns. For example: "what's wrong with me (her, him)—what can be done—will it be debilitating or fatal?" Family members both want answers and don't want them at the same time. Responses vary, from totally ignoring the condition and expecting the patient to function exactly as before, to a hand-wringing overconcern and oversolicitousness of every need of the patient. Either extreme is highly detrimental to family relationships. Ignoring the problem contributes to the patient's sense of having failed the family. It also often produces a desire in the patient to compensate by trying to do more than is physically or emotionally healthy, with potentially dire consequences. On the other hand, becoming overly involved with the patient may be infantilizing and can add to an already lowered self-esteem, and produce a slowly growing resentment in the family members.

A more healthy involvement of family members includes education, communication, and support. Most anxiety and reactions to the illness are the consequence of "not knowing." Family members should be as conversant with the patient's diagnosis, treatment, and prognosis as is the patient. Sharing of information between patient and family members is a necessity. This includes family members sharing their own feelings and concerns about whatever is on their minds, not just the illness. The patient may have a chronic illness, but is not helpless or incompetent. Being helpful to family members usually has a salutary effect upon patients. Finally, family members need to be involved in the illness itself, but only in ways that are useful from the patient's point of view. To do things for the patient, which he or she could do on his or her own, will frustrate the patient who has a need to be productive. To refuse to help, when the patient is helpless, will send a message that the family can't tolerate the illness. Family members need to distinguish these situations. Helping when help is truly needed, and backing off when it is not, are both kindnesses to the patient.

Looking back at these few paragraphs, one can notice how easy it is to focus on the patient's concerns. Family members need to be constantly aware of their own needs and concerns. Because the patient may not be able to contribute as in the past and family members may have to do more, family members need to program into their routine's time to "recharge their own batteries." Failure to do so will result in a growing resentment which will seep out in one's mannerisms, tone of voice, etc. —all to the detriment of family harmony.

It's important to remember that as family members, you count too. Your emotional comfort and well-being need just as much nurturing as do the patient's. In the long run, tending adequately to your own needs will make you a happier, more pleasant person to be with, and this is the best atmosphere for the growth of healthy family relationships.

FAMILIES MAKING ADJUSTMENTS

by Lawrence Kron, Ph.D.

Many of our readers will recognize the problem demonstrated by the following situation: A young mother, due to chronic illness, was required to make frequent trips to the hospital, sometimes two or three times in a year, for several weeks at a time. When her husband picked her up from the hospital, a consistent pattern of interaction between them emerged. No matter what the subject of their conversation, the husband would find reason to be critical of something or other, and an argument would follow.

At first we can only wonder, "What in the world is going on?" This should be a happy occasion, and yet the couple is in the middle of an argument before they have even reached their home. The explanation lies in understanding how families balance the roles they play in the family drama.

To some extent, every individual in a family is expected to take care of certain family responsibilities. The youngest member might be responsible for cleaning a bedroom. An older child might have responsibilities for dishes, shopping, etc. Mom might make meals. Dad may do some of the "fix it" tasks. In today's world, who assumes which tasks varies widely from one family to another. But however tasks are divided, everyone tends to be assigned a certain consistent role. You can imagine the chaos that would follow if there were no predictable roles. It would be like actors in a play suddenly being asked to play someone else's part. Yet, this is what happens in a family each time an exacerbation or a remission in a patient's illness occurs.

When a patient goes to the hospital, the rest of the family members have to do double duty, so to speak. They have to fill in for the missing member of the cast. They also need to take on new duties relating to the actual hospitalization demands. When the patient is sick enough to be taken to the hospital, our feelings of frustration are appropriately submerged. After all, "what right do we have to complain at a time like this?"

We do our best and adjust. But when the patient is feeling better and returns home, we again have to make an adjustment. It's difficult enough if everything returns to "normal." But even that is not always the case. The hospital routine may be replaced with a new routine for the home. The frustration of dealing with change once more rears its head. However, this time the patient is healthier. Our intuition tells us that we don't have to be as solicitous of the patient's feelings. The frustration of readjusting winds up being expressed by starting an argument.

Without realizing it, we are seeing the teeter-totter principle in action. If everyone is in perfect balance, we get upset with someone who changes position. We try to induce that person to remain in the place they occupied. If they don't, or can't, everyone else has to make a change in order to bring about a new balance. That changing of positions, of family roles, is what creates the problem I described above. It's my hope that by seeing the difficulty for what it is, you will be able to short-circuit the problem. If it should begin to occur in your family, instead of expressing your feelings indirectly, as was done by the husband I mentioned, perhaps you will be able to talk frankly with the patient about your concerns. The direct approach generally works best, and a great deal of heartache can be avoided.

GUILT
A FAMILY MEMBER'S PERSPECTIVE

by Lawrence Kron, Ph.D.

In the years that I've worked with the family members of patients with chronic illness, I've noticed how frequently they blame themselves in one way or another for the difficulties that the patient experiences. These feelings of guilt can be highly detrimental to family relationships. And they are rarely justified. Let's look at a few of the more common situations.

Parents often worry about the possibility of a genetic factor being involved in the onset of the illness in their children. Even when there is a hereditary predisposition, it is doubtful that heredity is the sole cause of the illness. And even if the illness is hereditary, how can we blame ourselves for something that we also inherited? The reality of this circumstance is that the patient and family members are all victims of bad luck.

Another form of guilt shows itself in the idea that a family member should not permit himself or herself to have fun if the patient cannot do so also. It is part of the "misery loves company" myth. If you, as a family member, deny yourself for this reason, you will most likely produce a sense of guilt or responsibility in the patient. Rather than helping to make the patient more comfortable, you will have added to the burdens of the illness.

Many family members have a sense of guilt because they feel well, and were lucky enough not to be stricken with the illness. I think of this as akin to "survivor guilt." In reality, everyone has to deal with the illness of a family member sooner or later. Would your family situation be improved if you also had a chronic illness? The family is actually lucky if only one member is ill. You can use the healthy energy you have to make adjustments in the family routine from time to time. This will enable the family to adjust most effectively to the ups and downs of the illness.

One of the more natural responses to dealing with a chronic illness in the family is a sense of frustration and resentment. Feeling guilty for having such reactions to the illness just adds fuel to the fire. Often the reactions occur because we have undertaken more tasks than the limitations of the illness require. There are many situations where the patient can help share some of the responsibilities. If you discuss your feelings with the patient, you will relieve some of your tensions in a more effective way. And, you will also avoid inducing a sense of guilt in him or her. You don't need an answer for every situation. Just speaking openly and honestly with the patient is often all that both of you need.

Often family members chastise themselves when the patient's illness flares up again. They ask, "What did I do to cause this? Could I or should I have acted differently in some way?" In an odd sort of way, we probably wish we were responsible. Then we would have the ability to change our behavior and positively affect the outcome of the illness. The truth is that many illnesses follow their own course, for the most part. There will be ups and downs, no matter what we do. We do know, however, that stress can create an environment in which chronic illness can flourish. We can do something if we help the patient to identify what is stressful for him or her. It is futile to try to guess what bothers a patient in every situation, and then attempt to avoid stress. Stress is highly individual and cannot be completely avoided. It's a matter of how we deal with it.* Each of us, patient and family member, have to do that for ourselves, but it also helps to be supportive of each other.

* *see letter on Stress*

Chapter Six

EMOTIONS IN CHRONIC ILLNESS

FEELINGS

Dear Audrey,

Since I have had my chronic illness, I have experienced so many different feelings that I'm beginning to wonder if I'm abnormal. Please let me know if others also experience mood swings. —P.G.

Dear P.G.,

Every human being experiences a wide range of feelings, all depending upon the circumstances. In fact, each day we encounter a variety of emotions. Certainly after the onset of an illness, it is quite common for one's emotions to be stirred up. Certain medicines may also cause mood swings. Each individual and each illness is different, but there are some strong feelings which we all share:

Fear. There may be fears about how the illness will affect work, school, or the future in general. Some of us worry that we will lose the love of our family and friends. Others are afraid of pain or the side effects from medication, hospitalization, and testing procedures.

Anger. "Why me?" is a common question. Sometimes the anger is directed against fate, but often it gets displaced to people we are close to and our family life is disrupted.

Guilt. Even though we might not know the specific cause of our illness, we often feel that we have done something to contribute to its onset. Even if that's not a concern, there may be guilty feelings for the extra burden that illness imposes on our family.

Shame. In our society we tend to think of people as healthy, strong, and often perfect. Television reinforces this view. Many people I've seen with a chronic illness come into therapy feeling that they are *flawed* in some way. It sometimes takes a while to turn the shame into pride at being able to deal with a chronic illness.

Depression. At times we feel like everything is going wrong. Life seems overwhelming, and it becomes difficult to believe that things will get better. We get down on ourselves and add to the burdens of the illness.

Frustration. Sometimes our bodies do not react in the way that we would like. We find we can't do everything we'd like. We become frustrated.

Alienation. There are times when we feel very isolated. It seems as if no one can understand what we are feeling.

It's important to recognize that all of these feelings are perfectly normal and commonly experienced. If we acknowledge our emotions, we will be able to talk to others about them. This is an important part of the process of learning to accept them.

EMBARRASSMENT

Dear Audrey,

I have a chronic illness and I am often so embarrassed. I was wondering if there was anything you could suggest to help me get through these difficult times. —S.B.

Dear S.B.,

Those of us who live with chronic illnesses often experience some types of embarrassment. You didn't mention what was embarrassing you, but there are many situations that could cause these feelings. Some people are embarrassed because their looks are altered from medication, or as a result of the illness. Others are embarrassed because they are limited in what they can do or eat. Some are embarrassed because they are incontinent. It could be seizures for someone with epilepsy, lack of motor control in Parkinson's disease or multiple sclerosis, or the unexpected verbalizations caused by Tourette Syndrome.

Some individuals are embarrassed because they have to use a wheelchair or need some other type of equipment. There are a multitude of circumstances which can make individuals with a chronic illness feel different. Let me offer some suggestions that may help you minimize embarrassment.

- **Plan ahead**. Think of the potential circumstances for embarrassment, and learn to take steps to avert them. Inform those closest to you what they have to do. Carry instructions for emergency situations. Try to picture the worst possible situation, and then think of what you can do to offset it. Prepare what you might say in the worst possible situation. You may not be witty in the midst of a disaster, but you can certainly work on some choice comments to ease a situation. If you can't think of anything clever, at least think about it in advance so you still have time to ask others for their ideas.

- **Remember; you haven't done anything to be ashamed of**. In fact, you should be proud that you are able to handle the challenge of a chronic illness. It takes a special person to adjust to the demands of living with illness.

- **Put the focus on your other attributes**. You are more than just your illness. Do the best you can to accentuate your character strength and your appearance. Develop meaningful friendships. Good friends are less likely to be put off by the embarrassing features of your illness. They will be concentrating on your positive qualities. For additional help, review the letter on "Making Friends."

- **Talk to a friend** about how the embarrassing situation felt to you. Just talking and being listened to can be very healing.

- **Put an embarrassing incident in perspective**. Even people without chronic illness have embarrassing moments. Although it is sometimes difficult, remind yourself that most embarrassing situations are soon forgotten by everybody. Don't you be the one to hold onto them. Think how unimportant they will be next year, next week or even an hour from now.

- **Ask yourself, "What can I learn from this**?" Life's embarrassments often teach us humility or empathy. They teach us how to be strong so that we can deal with whatever life throws our way in the future.

- **Try to develop a sense of humor**. If you can laugh at a situation, it puts others at ease. Most people are uncomfortable because they aren't sure what you are feeling.

When you do find yourself in the middle of an embarrassing situation, just stop for a minute and develop a plan of action. Recently, I was at a bridal shower, and as I headed for the bathroom, the clip on my ostomy came off. I wanted to just sit down and cry, but I knew that wouldn't help. I quickly went into the bathroom and cleaned myself off. I gathered some paper towels and cleaned up the mess on the floor. I was able to pull myself together in time to say good-bye to the hostess and bride.

From this incident I learned I had to be more careful with my clip, and that I must not wait so long to go to the bathroom. I also kept telling myself that I've gotten through worse and that I was doing the best that I could.

So, S.B., I know there will be times you might feel embarrassed by your chronic illness, and that isn't pleasant. But, it's important to remember that you are not just your illness. Become a person you can be proud of. If you feel this is overwhelming, get professional help. Because when you are proud of yourself, embarrassments will become incidental.

FORGIVENESS

Dear Audrey,

I am so angry at my mother for how she treated me when I was a child. Now my therapist is telling me that my health would improve if I could forgive her. I also feel that with all she did to me, I have the right not to forgive her. I don't know what forgiveness has to do with my illness. I wondered if you had some thoughts about the connection. —F.S.

Dear F. S.,

Many people with chronic illnesses harbor grudges from the past. Unfortunately, the one that is hurt is the individual who carries the resentment, not the individual who is blamed for the problem. Long-term anger and resentment have a way of wearing down your system and keeping your body from healing.

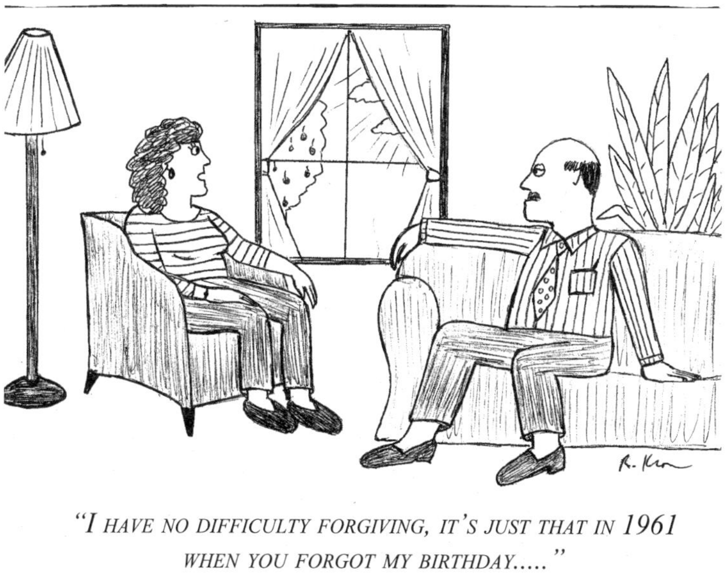

"I HAVE NO DIFFICULTY FORGIVING, IT'S JUST THAT IN 1961 WHEN YOU FORGOT MY BIRTHDAY....."

Often one thinks that forgiveness means forgetting, condoning, or giving in, and that makes it difficult to accept. Forgiveness is actually a healing process. It is realizing that attempting to punish people from our past will not heal us. It is valuing ourselves enough to let go of the intense feelings from the past, moving beyond our grudges and resentments.

In their book, *Forgiveness,** Dr. Sidney Simon and Suzanne Simon note the following stages of forgiveness:

- Denial, when we tend to play down the significance of events in our past.

- Self blame, when we blame ourselves for what happened.

- Victim, when we recognize the hurt, feel we didn't deserve it, and wallow in self-pity.

- Indignation, when we are angry and self-righteous, and we want the people whom we believe hurt us to suffer.

- Survival, when we recognize that we were hurt, and we did survive. We become aware of our strengths, develop a sense of humor and realize that we did the best that we could.

- Integration, when we accept that those that we blame for hurting us may have been doing the best they could. "If we are more than our wounds, they must be more than the inflictors of those wounds ... we can put the past in perspective ... without forgetting it ... let go of the pain, and get on with our lives unencumbered by excess emotional baggage."

It is certainly important for you to work through the stages of your healing. Your therapist can help you, and you may speed the process with the book I mentioned.

* *see Appendix 2*

The method you choose is up to you. However, holding on to your grudges will probably be detrimental to your health. We don't know the causes of many diseases, but we do know that aggravation plays a part in exacerbations. Holding on to past resentments is not conducive to getting well.

Seek help to guide you through the stages of forgiveness, and get on with your life. Your body has a better chance to heal when energy isn't being wasted on resentment of past injustices.

ACCEPTANCE

Dear Audrey,

I was diagnosed three months ago. I can't accept my illness, and I can't deal with it. My friend told me to write to you. I don't think it can help, but I said I would. —G.J.

Dear G. J.,

You really sound hopeless and helpless. I can understand that hearing you have a chronic illness is overwhelming. However, in time, most people adjust quite well and learn to lead a fairly normal life with some modifications. But it is difficult in the beginning. Let me offer some suggestions to help you get past this hopeless feeling.

Don't be too harsh on yourself. In the beginning just the knowledge that you have a chronic illness is a loss; it is a loss of your old healthy self and some mourning is normal.

Get informed. I am assuming that you have taken the steps necessary to determine that you have a correct diagnosis. If there is any doubt, get another opinion.

If you're sure your diagnosis is correct and the helpless and hopeless feelings persist, it's time to start taking control. Get all the information you can. Chronic illness organizations* have many excellent books and pamphlets available. There are also tapes you can listen to and meetings to attend which will help increase your understanding of your illness. Once you have a greater understanding of what your illness is and how to live successfully with it, you will feel much more accepting of it.

With information and experience, you will learn ways to handle situations that now seem oppressive. For most problems there are solutions. It's just a matter of spending time to find them.

Get a good health-care team. Ask around. Call your local hospitals. Ask for recommendations from your particular chronic illness organization, or anyone you know who has your illness or knows of someone dealing with it. You need a doctor with whom you can work comfortably. You may need a nutritionist, a home health care organization, or a therapist. Don't hesitate to enlist any support that is available.

Along with the support of health-care professionals, you will need a solid personal support system. Even though it may be difficult, keeping in contact with friends and family is very important. You might also enlist the aid of a chronic illness support group.

Alter your attitude. It will be helpful if you list all the positive things in your life. If you concentrate, you will see much that is easy to take for granted. Consider the people you know. Are there loved ones, friends, religious advisors, teachers, health care professionals, who have helped you? If you find this task terribly difficult, as can happen when you get very depressed, you may want to get professional help from a therapist.

Let up on yourself. I have found that many people I work with who have chronic illnesses, are perfectionists. Having the illness keeps them from living life as they feel they "should." Getting rid of the "shoulds" can make life much easier.

* *see Appendix 1*

Try to make the most of the challenges you face. Your life will be much more gratifying if you accept having the illness, and then see how best you can handle it.

It's tremendously important to accept what you can't change so that you can use your energy to make changes that are possible.

Finally, many people find that therapy is very helpful.

WHEN IS THERAPY APPROPRIATE?

Dear Audrey,
My doctor suggested that I go into group therapy. She feels it will help my chronic illness. I wonder if therapy is appropriate for chronic illness, or would a support group be sufficient? —H.Z.

Dear H.Z.,
As we know, living with a chronic illness can add stress to our lives. Many chronic illness organizations have developed support groups that are not professionally led. These mutual help groups can provide a very helpful support network for patients and their families. However, some situations may require more than a support group. Then therapy should be considered.

Some questions you may want to ponder are:

Why would a person with a chronic illness want therapy?

The burdens of daily living can at times seem overwhelming. Adding the burden of chronic illness contributes to the stress. One purpose of therapy is to help us respond to stressful situations more effectively, and thereby ease the burden.

Another purpose of therapy is to help identify what is the real stressor, and why it is so stressful. Becoming more self aware is a powerful tool in coping with chronic illness. We know that stress affects the immune system, and many illnesses are connected to the immune system. Therapy is also a way to regain some control of our life when the chronic illness makes us feel so out of control.

What are the concerns of people with chronic illness?

Some of the more common concerns relate to diet, medication, financial burdens, insurance complications, pain, hospitalization, surgery, tests, loss and the uncertainty of the illness. Some people are concerned about the possibility of dying. Added to this list are many interpersonal concerns, such as how the illness affects relationships with family and friends, or conditions at work and school, or how one feels about oneself.

Is stress the same for everybody?

No. What is stressful for one person may not be for another. Sometimes we are not even aware that something is stressful unless we explore it further.

Why would therapy benefit people with chronic illness? Doesn't everybody have to deal with stress?

Yes, and it would be helpful for everyone to learn more effective ways to deal with life's stresses. Those with chronic illness need to learn to manage the stress of everyday life, and that's complicated by the stress of the illness. In addition, the consequences for people with chronic illness can be more severe, at times making the physical problems worse. Therefore managing stress becomes more crucial.

Why is group therapy often recommended?

A group offers the unique opportunity to share feelings with others who have also experienced the problems associated with chronic illness. It helps a person feel less alone. It provides an opportunity to see how others cope. Sometimes others can express feelings that you have experienced, but may not have been able to articulate. There is also the satisfaction of being able to help others. A group helps alter distorted self images and can furnish hope. In addition, groups deal with areas of concern in a safe environment, giving the skills and insight to be able to apply these methods in the "outside" world. This safe environment is also conducive to the expression of feelings that are better let out than held in, where they could possibly exacerbate the illness.

Regardless of whether it's by self examination, reading, talking, support groups, or individual or group therapy, taking care of your emotional well-being is an important part of your total health care.

Chapter Seven

COPING TECHNIQUES

DEALING WITH STRESS

Dear Audrey,

I hear so much about stress being bad for chronic illnesses. But this is such a stressful world! How can I possibly avoid stress? —I.S.

Dear I. S.,

You are right about stress being bad for chronic illness. Stress affects the immune system, and the immune system has a direct relationship to many chronic illnesses. Problems with the immune system can prevent necessary healing. However, you cannot avoid all stress, nor would you want to. A certain amount of stress is healthy.

If we didn't have some stress, we wouldn't get out of the way when a car comes toward us. We need stress to just get out of bed in the morning. What is important to avoid is too much stress. And yes, we do live in a stressful world. Someone recently said that today, if you have children, you can't avoid stress. Wars, economic problems, natural disasters, crime, illness, and even traffic all lead to stress. We need to learn how to cope with it and to find ways to alleviate the excess.

I'm going to give you a list of "stress busters." Think of them like a wardrobe. You don't have to use them all at once, and different ones will be appropriate for different situations. If you have a closet full of clothes or a repertoire of stress busters, you will be prepared for whatever circumstance arises.

Throughout this book, I have mentioned various ways of coping with stress. Some of the methods I mention elsewhere are:

- Identifying the problem and making sure you know exactly what it is that you need to address.

- Working on yourself instead of trying to change other people.

- Maintaining realistic expectations of others to avoid disappointment.
- Finding a way you can gain control of a difficult situation.
- Learning time-management techniques.
- Remembering, if nothing else, you can always change your attitude or the way you look at a particular incident.
- Gaining information.
- Finding a support system.
- Using laughter.

Here are some additional ways to deal with stress that may also work in different instances.

Nurture connections with others.

- Accept that others are different and have the right to be.
- Make love, not war. Sex is a good stress reliever.
- Talk to a friend.
- Express your feelings. Make sure it's someone who wants to listen.
- Work on your listening skills.

Take care of your body.

- Cut down on coffee and colas containing caffeine.
- Walk it off. A ten or fifteen-minute walk can be very effective.
- Take a hot bath.
- Take time to do just nothing.
- Try for some form of daily exercise to increase your sense of well-being.
- Get enough sleep and rest. Consult your doctor if you have trouble sleeping.
- Listen to your body rhythms. If you are a morning person, do the hardest jobs in the morning.
- Avoid self-medication. Drugs and alcohol might mask the symptoms, but they won't help you deal with the stress.

- Understand the medicines you are taking and how they should be used.
- Become an expert on nutrition. There is no one perfect diet for all chronic illnesses. However, it is important that you establish a nutritional diet that agrees with you. This can take a lot of trial and error because diets vary for everyone and can even vary for the same individual at different stages of the illness. It is worth the trouble it takes. A well-nourished body can help you deal with stress.
- Find a doctor in whom you have confidence and to whom you can relate.
- Consider getting training in yoga, meditation or relaxation techniques.
- Get your emotional life together. Don't forget that the mind and the body work together. If something is bothering you emotionally, it can affect your body.

Increase interests and fun level in your life.

- Listen to your favorite music.
- Take vacations. They can just be a weekend close by. The important part is changing your regular routine and concentrating on having fun.
- Find a hobby you enjoy. Try not to get into the TV rut, an easy thing to do when you are stuck in bed. Look at the TV schedule and tune in or tape only the programs that you especially enjoy.
- Have more fun. You may even need help deciding what is fun for you.

Become more informed.

- Read some psychology self-help books. I have listed some in Appendix two, and the library and bookstores have many more. It would take you a lifetime to read all the material written about stress.
- Find role-models to inspire you. Biographies of people who have dealt with your problems can be a rich source of inspiration.

- Call your illness support group* and get all the information about your illness that you can.

Organize your life.

- Prioritize and put things in perspective.
- Build in an extra half hour cushion time for daily events and an extra day for large projects. You will then have time to deal with the unexpected and not feel stressed.
- Learn to say "no."
- Take frequent breaks from work at the office or home.
- Write notes to help you remember. Keep a date book, and keep all your notes together.
- Take care of as much as you can as you go along. It's very stressful when things build up. Something as simple as handling each piece of paper only once and taking care of it can make a big difference.
- Keep your car and household appliances in good condition. Avoid stress of unexpected breakdowns.
- Change some aspects of your daily routine. For instance, sleep on the opposite side of the bed; vary your dressing routine; eat something different than you usually do. (You don't have to be rigid to be organized.)
- Make life as convenient as possible. For instance, acquire advance information on the physical layout of places you are visiting. Will they be barrier free if that is a requirement for you? How much walking will you have to do? Is there a more convenient way of entering the building?

Change your attitude.

- Don't sweat "small stuff." (Most problems are "small stuff.")
- Appreciate what you do have.
- Change what you can, accept what you can't and know the difference.

* *see Appendix 1*

- Appreciate the NOW.
- It's not perfect to be perfect: Let go of "shoulds." One of my groups gave me permission to share their "Eleventh Commandment: Thou shalt not 'should' thyself to death."
- Instead of automatically saying, "I can't do it," try and find a way to adapt.
- Clear your conscience. What has happened to you is not a punishment. As Harold Kushner teaches us, "bad things do happen to good people.*"
- Help someone else. It will get your mind off yourself.
- Don't give up hope.

I hope that these suggestions will help you cope more effectively with stress. As you read through the rest of the book, you will find many other ways to help keep stress in your life to a minimum.

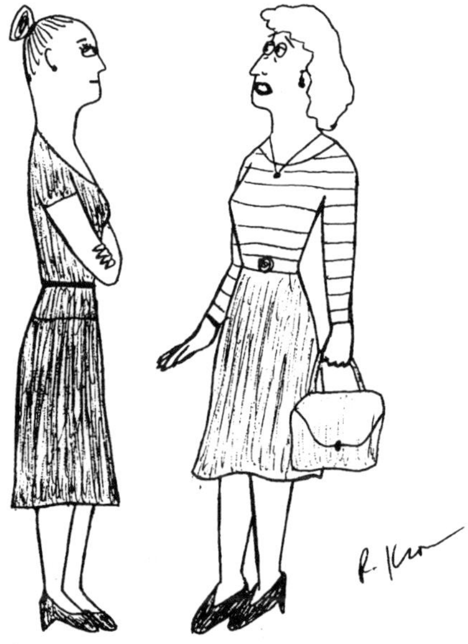

I ATTENDED A STRESS MANAGEMENT WORKSHOP, AND NOW I WORRY MORE EFFECTIVELY.

* *see Appendix 2*

LAUGHING

Dear Audrey,

My neighbor told me that laughter can be helpful for my illness and I was furious. She should know that this disease is no laughing matter. Where did she ever get that idea? —S.S.

Dear S.S.,

I certainly agree with you that chronic illness is not a laughing matter; however, let's not discount the value of laughter. A great deal of research is being done on the effects of laughter on the immune system. Norman Cousins popularized this theory when he literally laughed his way to health. He helped cure himself of a serious illness by watching humorous TV programs and putting himself on a regular regimen of laughing. I'm not saying that laughter could cure your illness. Don't we wish it could? However, laughter provides many benefits. For instance, when you laugh, your cardiovascular system dilates so the rate of blood flow increases.

According to Annette Goodheart,* "the laughter lady," on her audiotape entitled, *Laugh Your Way to Health*, "It's like internal jogging. Your muscles go slack. You lose control." She goes on to say that many of us are afraid of losing control. That's unfortunate because, after a good belly laugh, the brain releases a powerful pain killing substance called beta endorphin which is 100 times more powerful than any morphine-type drug you can take. Haven't you noticed that your pain is substantially reduced, if not gone entirely, for the short time just after you've had a good laugh? Once we can see the value of laughter, our next step is to determine how we can add more laughter to our lives. Here are a few suggestions. Once you get started, more will come to you.

**Dr. Annette Goodheart can be reached at:*
P.O. Box 40297
Santa Barbara, CA 03140-0297

- Keep a collection of articles, stories, jokes, — items that make you laugh.
- Get comedy tapes and records from the library.
- Look for the humor in situations.
- Don't be afraid to be silly.
- If possible, attend a conference on laughter and play.*
- Put cartoons with funny sayings up on the refrigerator door, the office bulletin board or even in the bathroom.

One of the nicest aspects of laughter is that there are no side effects. It doesn't have to cost anything. It unites people, and it's just plain fun. Our symptoms can all be more tolerable if we bring some laughter to them, no matter how hard that seems. Jules Feiffer says: "You've got to laugh at yourself sometimes. If you can't climb the mountain of yourself head-on, you've got to find a flight of stairs that no one had discovered before. Those stairs can be humor."

I know you are not happy with your illness, but remember the comment attributed to William James: "We don't laugh because we're happy, we're happy because we laugh."

**For more information about conferences on laughter and play write:*

The Humor Project at Saratoga Institute
110 Spring St.
Saratoga Springs, NY 12866
(518)587-8770

The Institute for the Advancement of Human Behavior
(The Power of Laughter and Play Conference)
P.O. Box 7226
Stanford, CA 94309
FAX (415) 851-0406

RETAINING RESPONSIBILITY:

Dear Audrey,

I was looking forward to becoming an officer of our P.T.A., but I was not nominated because one of my friends said that because I had a chronic illness it might be too difficult for me. I was so disappointed. How would you handle this situation? —S.W.

Dear Audrey,

I recently applied for a job and asked one of my friends for a letter of reference. I accidentally found out that he had written that he didn't think that I would be able to handle the job because of my chronic illness. I'm really frustrated about this. Do you have any suggestions? —H.H.

Dear Audrey,

Since I was diagnosed with a chronic illness, I notice that my family is not sharing family issues with me. My daughter was having some difficulty, and she didn't even let me know. I really feel left out. Could you address this matter? —T.L.

Dear Audrey,

My friends feel that social activities will be too draining for me, so consequently I haven't been asked to any parties, concerts, etc. I know that sometimes I can't go, but it feels so lonely to not even be asked. Please put this letter in your column to let the public know that we don't want to be excluded because we have a chronic illness. —C.D.

I have condensed these letters and grouped them together because they all deal with a difficult problem which those of us with a chronic illness face. Often our family and friends feel that they are being helpful by protecting us. What they don't realize is that they are diminishing us as individuals by not letting us make decisions for ourselves.

Sometimes others feel that because we are having physical problems, that we are intellectually compromised as well. It's important to explain to family and friends that we want to retain our autonomy. Regardless of whether we can or cannot do something, we should be consulted on matters affecting our lives.

However, if we expect others to consult with us, we, too, have to take some responsibility. We have to let others know what we can do and how we plan on doing it. We have to learn to say no to requests we feel we cannot handle and find adaptive ways to deal with the obligations that we do undertake. Talk with the significant people in your life and let them know that you want the option of making your own decisions. Let them know that this is very important to you.

FINDING ADVANTAGES

Dear Audrey,

A woman at work had the audacity to tell me that in many ways she found a chronic illness to be helpful. I was furious at first. My illness is definitely not helpful to me. However, when I calmed down, I decided to write to you and see if you had any ideas about her comment. —I.W.

Dear I.W.

I can understand that having a chronic illness is difficult enough without unsolicited opinions from others. However, your question made me ponder the concept. Is there anything helpful about having a chronic illness?

As funny as it may seem, there actually are some benefits; what some call secondary gains. An example might be those unpleasant situations we can avoid because we are sick. Or perhaps we gain extra attention. However, I wouldn't really call these secondary gains helpful. The illness is too big a price to pay.

However, if we think about it, there really are some positive aspects to having a chronic illness. Some of the advantages I have found are as follows:

It certainly makes us appreciate the times when we are feeling well. Others go through life taking it for granted. We learn to value each day.

It presents a challenge to help us grow. It pushes us to go beyond our comfort zone and learn to handle more difficult situations. This helps us to become stronger people.

It gives us a better understanding of others who face difficulties in their lives.

If we work at it, we can make our relationships stronger. People who struggle through problems together become even closer.

It may influence our career. In my case, having Crohn's disease was an important part of why I became a psychotherapist. I went back to school so that I could work with people struggling with chronic illness. I have heard of others who became doctors, nurses, nutritionists, or sales representatives for drug companies.

We become part of an international network of people with our illness. Through our own respective organizations, we meet people and become involved in a meaningful endeavor: we work to find the cure and to help others. And we also may make new friends in the process.

So, I.W., I'm glad you sought an opinion. You gave us all an opportunity to consider some of the helpful aspects of the illness.

CHANGING ATTITUDES

Dear Readers,

One of the problems many of us share is that we have unrealistic expectations. We have enough to contend with in dealing with the illness, but then we put unnecessary additional stress on our lives. Albert Ellis* called some of these expectations "irrational ideas."

I'll share with you a few of these "irrational ideas," which are the source of many coping difficulties. The sooner we realize that they are irrational, the sooner we can get on with coping.

- First, there's the idea that it is a dire necessity for an adult human being to be loved or approved of by virtually every significant other person in his community.

- Second, there's the idea that one should be thoroughly competent, adequate, and achieving in all possible respects, if one is to consider oneself worthwhile. (This is an idea we see often.)

- Third, is the idea that it is awful and catastrophic when things are not the way one would very much like them to be.

- Fourth, is the idea that it is easier to avoid than to face certain life difficulties and self responsibilities.

- Fifth, is the idea that one should be dependent on others and that one needs someone stronger than oneself on whom to rely.

- Finally, there is the idea that there is invariably a right, precise, and perfect solution to human problems, and that it is catastrophic if this perfect solution is not found.

*Ellis, Albert, *A New Guide to Rational Living.*

We can surely see how harboring some of these beliefs can be detrimental to our health. Let us hope that we can recognize them, address them, and eventually eliminate this needless source of stress. High expectations are admirable, but keep them rational.

FEELING ISOLATED

Dear Audrey,

I live in a very small town where there are no support groups for my particular illness. I am sure there are others with my illness somewhere, but I don't know any of them. I feel so isolated. Do you have any suggestions? —W.L.

Dear W.L.,

Find the nearest town in which there is an appropriate support group for you. (There is a list at the back of this book.) Even if the closest chapter is quite far away, you can get on the mailing list, and plan to attend some special events. A coping conference or contact with a support group will be helpful in reducing your feelings of loneliness.

You might even want to start a chapter or a support group in your area. Ask your doctor if he can put you in touch with others who would be interested. Contact either your closest chapter or the national office for guidelines. Whatever you do, you will want to join (or to create) a chapter that you can become involved with. The American Clearing House,* can be helpful in either case.

Read everything you can. In Appendix Two, I list some books that give a greater understanding of chronic illness. Meanwhile, check with the most convenient office of your particular illness organization and see what is available there in books and pamphlets.

* *see Appendix 1*

You might consider corresponding with someone who shares your circumstances. Sometimes just having someone listen to you can be beneficial. Find a friend who wants to listen, or consult with a member of the clergy. If they are not knowledgeable about your illness, you can educate them with the available literature.

You might also talk to a therapist who is familiar with your illness. Even if there is no one available in your town, there are some therapists who now do phone consultations regardless of how far away you live. Again, your local or national chronic illness organization should have this information.

Whichever way you proceed, it is important to make some connections with others who understand the effects of the illness.

INDEPENDENT THINKING

Dear Audrey,

Would you please expand on the phrase "independent thinking" referred to in your column, and include the various outlets our own inner resources can furnish us to connect with life, though we may be occasionally forced into a sedentary position? —D.T.

Dear D.T.,

It is frustrating enough to have a chronic illness, but it adds insult to injury when others feel that, because our body is weak, our mind is also weak. Often when we are hospitalized, the nurses talk to us as if we have a child's mentality and are completely dependent. "Now we will take our bath," is a classic example. Unfortunately, after awhile we buy into the idea that because at times we are dependent physically, we are also dependent mentally. That couldn't be further from the truth. *One of the most independent men I have ever known was flat on his back and unable to move.* He had

Amyotrophic Lateral Sclerosis, but that didn't stop him from using his mind in order to lead a life of dignity.

Here are some ways to nurture this independent thinking—ways that don't require much physical energy.

- First of all there is always the wonderful postal system, E-mail, and the fax machine. They enable you to get involved in politics, correspond with someone in a foreign land, reach out to others, and in many ways, connect with the outside world.

- Today, the outside world is brought to you through radio, television, books, magazines, tapes and computers. Being flat on your back is no excuse for not keeping up with what's happening in the world. Find interesting topics to talk about. Read, listen, watch. Participate!

- Don't shut out your friends because you can't run with them. Invite them to visit. Refreshments can be ordered in or brought by your friends. Be inventive. Serve picnic-style, using disposable plates and flatware to make things easier.

- Write about your experiences by keeping a journal. You don't have to be professional. Years later, these journal entries will be enlightening.

- Learn something new. For example, you can learn a language through tapes or records.

- Use the phone. Not only can you keep up your social contacts, but you can also utilize the phone to run your house or business. Even in a sedentary position, with the aid of a phone you can shop, secure services, obtain information, and accomplish many of the tasks that you previously did in person.

- Pursue your existing hobbies or find new ones.

- If you are a parent unable to participate in active sports with your children, read to them or play games as an alternative means of connecting.

- Reach out to others through the use of a personal computer. Through the Internet you can access all corners of the world. In some cases, you can even get information about your disease, and talk to others with common concerns.

- Remember, just because your body is weak doesn't mean you can't take part in family decisions and offer emotional support.

- Become a home-based volunteer. Many organizations can use volunteers at home for calling or writing. This is an ideal way to help others as you help yourself.

Remember; you have a *chronic* illness. Although you will have difficult periods, there are also periods when you can get out and enjoy life. With a good sense of humor, an inquiring mind, and a little creativity, even the most difficult periods of your life can be meaningful.

BECOMING MORE ASSERTIVE

Dear Audrey,

I never was very assertive, and now since I've been sick I feel like I've lost all power. I'm always doing things I don't want to do and frequently feel that nobody is paying attention to what I say. The whole situation is very depressing, and I would appreciate any help. It's hard enough handling these problems when I am feeling well, but with my illness it seems impossible. —G.C.

Dear G.C.,

I have found that not being assertive is not only depressing in and of itself, but it also can contribute to making your illness worse. Individuals who end up doing more than they want and not feeling that they have any power, tend to feel resentful. Not speaking up results in the resentment going inside to do more damage to an already vulnerable body. So I'm glad that you were assertive enough to write for some help.

First of all, let us be sure that we agree on what assertiveness is. Many people confuse being aggressive with being assertive. Being assertive is standing up for our rights; being aggressive is violating the rights of others. There are many ways to be assertive. We might just state our needs, feelings or opinions. But, it often helps to recognize the other person's needs first. For example we might say, "I can understand that you want me to take this medicine, but I need to know the side effects."

Many individuals with chronic illness have a hard time saying "no." Perhaps they feel that they have to make up for having a chronic illness. Or perhaps they have learned as children that what they want isn't important, or that confronting others is not acceptable. Whatever the reason, saying "yes" all the time is not a good solution. If you say "yes" and mean it, you may take on too much work and wear yourself out. If you say "yes" just because it is easier to say than "no"— even if you don't really mean it you will have to deal with the anger and disappointment of others when you don't follow through. Thus it is important to learn to say "no."

Sometimes this may be accomplished by simply saying "no." At other times you might want to explain your response. At times that may be too difficult for you. Then you can refuse part of the request and state what you can do. Or you might offer the person an alternative. If you are still having difficulty, a good book to consult is, *When I Say No I Feel Guilty*.*

Another way to stand up for your rights is to just say, "I understand that you feel. . . .but I feel ..." Keep repeating the same statement. Eventually the person will realize you are not going to back down. If speaking up continues

* *see Appendix 2*

to be a problem, consider different ways to become more comfortable expressing your feelings. One way is to write your ideas out ahead of time. Rehearsing what you want to communicate with a friend or counselor ahead of time can also make you feel more confident.

As a patient it is possible to be assertive in many ways. Just because you have a chronic illness doesn't mean you have to lose all your power. You need to establish a relationship with your health care professionals which makes you one of the team. Gaining information, asking questions and reading about your illness all add to your empowerment. Doing what you can for yourself and being able to ask for help when it is needed, also adds to your strength.

If you are having difficulty becoming assertive, refer to the excellent books I have listed in Appendix 2. You might also consider an assertiveness training class. There are many available at schools or hospitals. If you are still having difficulty, you might want to get professional help. A skilled therapist can determine if you have trouble asserting yourself because you feel unworthy, need to be punished, have had traumatic childhood experiences, or are dealing with other issues.

But, please, G.C., take the next step and act so that you can become more assertive. Not only will you be happier, but you will probably be healthier.

VOLUNTEERING

Dear Audrey,

Recently I had surgery, and I'm feeling well enough to get around, but I don't feel ready to get back to work. I'm bored staying home. Do you have any suggestions? —R.G.

Dear R.G.,

Your situation is very common — the uncomfortable middleground of being too well to be home, and not well enough to handle the pressures of work. I have a suggestion that will be helpful not only for you, but for others as well. Think about doing volunteer work. Your local support group* would be a perfect place to begin. Start in a capacity in which you feel comfortable. Here are some of the numerous advantages:

- You will feel useful.
- You will be performing a needed service.
- You will meet people.
- You will be in an atmosphere where people understand what you are going through.
- You will learn more about your illness.
- You can use this experience in your resume when you return to work.
- You can build up your strength in a stress-free situation.
- You will learn new skills.
- You will have structure in your day that is not overwhelming.

Getting dressed, getting out, and accepting some responsibility may seem difficult at first. However, you will feel better when you do. Take advantage of this opportunity.

PONDERING THOUGHTS ON HAPPINESS

Dear Readers,

I recently found some information on happiness and thought I would share it with you. Finding happiness despite chronic illness requires a whole repertoire of ideas on which to draw. Several years ago the sociology depart-

* *see Appendix 1*

ment at Duke University did a study called "Peace of Mind." Several factors were found to contribute greatly to emotional and mental stability. They are:

- The absence of suspicion and resentment. Nursing a grudge was a major factor in unhappiness.

- Living in the present rather than the past. An unwholesome preoccupation with old mistakes and failures leads to depression.

- Accepting what cannot be changed, rather than wasting time and energy fighting conditions outside of your control.

- Cooperating with life, instead of trying to run away from it.

- Forcing oneself to stay involved with the world, and resisting the temptation to withdraw and become reclusive during periods of emotional stress.

- Refusing to indulge in self-pity when life hands you a raw deal and accepting the fact that nobody gets through life without some sorrow and misfortune.

- Cultivating old-fashioned virtues: love, honor, compassion, and loyalty.

- Having realistic expectations. Don't expect too much of yourself. When there is too wide a gap between self-expectation and your ability to meet the goals you have set, feelings of inadequacy are inevitable.

- Finding something bigger than yourself to believe in. Self-centered, egotistical people score lowest in any test for measuring happiness.

As you look over these factors, I hope they will give you some ideas on how you can improve the quality of your life.

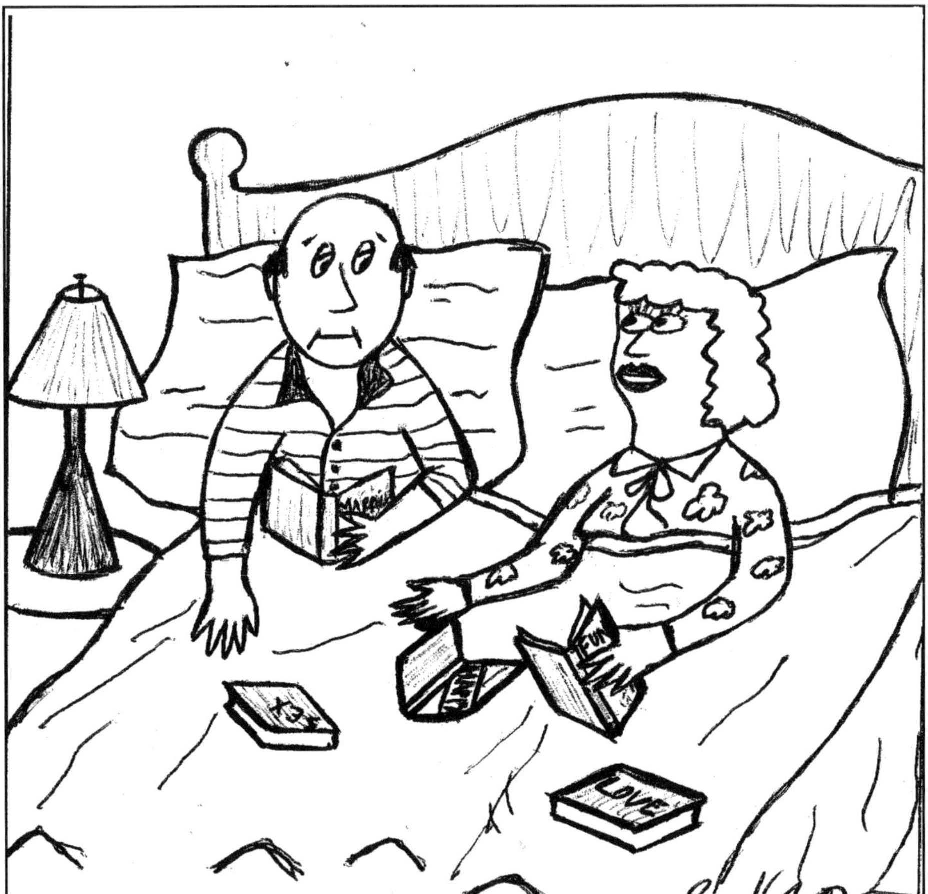

ARE WE HAPPY YET?

READING

Dear Audrey,

I have always found that reading was very helpful for me. Do you have anything that you would recommend to make dealing with my chronic illness any easier? —N.R.

Dear N.R.,

I applaud your search for reading material. Those that read certainly have a head start in the coping arena. Finding new information is a very important aspect of coping.

In the second appendix I have included a list of books I think will be helpful. Not only have I included books on many aspects of coping with chronic illness, but I have also included books that deal with other areas which I feel will improve the quality of your life. Unfortunately, there are only a small number of books available dealing with chronic illness in general. I listed all I could find. I did not include the many books on individual chronic illnesses. There are some very good books that deal with specific illnesses. If you contact the support organization for your illness,* they can help you find books on your particular illness. In many cases they will also have some literature for you which is either free, or available for a minimal charge.

I have also listed books on the mind-body connection and stress. These books point out the connection between stress and illness and offer ways to help you deal with the stress. Stress plays an important part in all illness. I'm not saying it causes your illness, although there are some illnesses that are directly related to stress. But there is growing evidence that once you have an illness, stress must be considered. It often causes an exacerbation of symptoms or hinders the healing process. What makes it more difficult is that chronic illness itself is stressful. All of us with a chronic illness can benefit from knowing more about the mind-body connection.

**see Appendix 1*

I have included books about relationships, because even good relationships are affected by chronic illness, and most of us can use some help to keep our relationships healthy. Having a good relationship can be a very important part of the healing process.

I have also included some information on parenting, but you might search out additional books on this topic. New books appear all the time. Parenting is difficult enough, but if you or your spouse has a chronic illness, there is more pressure on you as parents. If you have a child with a chronic illness, additional skills are required as well.

There are many books available on improving the quality of life in general. Look in the self-help section of book stores or libraries. Anything that helps you become a stronger, happier person can only make coping with your illness easier. I have suggested a few titles to get you started.

The inspirational books are included for days when life seems too tough. At those times we can benefit from learning how others have met their difficult challenges or have developed a useful philosophy.

I have also included a few humorous books at the end. Humor is *very* important. Browse through your library or bookstore in the humor section. See what appeals to you. You'll have no trouble finding a vast array of books that will help you laugh.

I am not endorsing everything in every book, but they can give you some fresh ideas and help you form your own coping strategies. Finding these titles will lead you to the right section in the library or bookstore. Once there, stop and browse. A day in the library or bookstore in itself is very comforting. Don't forget that used bookstores may also have some of the selections at reduced prices. Also check out the books on tape for the days when you don't even have the energy to read. Some libraries will mail you books or books on tape if you are housebound because of your illness. Also if your library does not have the books you are looking for, don't hesitate to ask. They may be able to get the book from another library, or in some cases, order a copy.

Keep reading. Remember; good reading can be a gateway to good health.

AFTERWORD: LIFE IS UNCERTAIN

MORE CRISES, MORE CHALLENGES

Earlier I had indicated that with a chronic illness there is a concern that the frequency of the various episodes of the illness soon becomes boring. I had finished "My Story" part of this book and was content to leave it where it was. However my most recent encounter with the challenge of chronic illness has taught me new lessons that I also want to share with you, my readers. So now, let me describe the events of the last month. I want you to know what happened, but more importantly, I want you to know what I learned from them.

With a chronic illness, life often seems like a roller coaster. Everything seemed to be going well for me, and then my pain became unbearable and Dr. Diokno suspected that kidney stones were the culprits. He told me over the phone that he wanted me in the hospital immediately. I had time to throw a few items in a suitcase and left for the hospital. Originally I had thought that I would be able to see a client on my way to the hospital, but quickly realized that would be impossible. My husband and I drove to the office and I told the client that I would call her as soon as I knew what was happening. She too was suffering from a chronic illness. My cancellation had been therapeutic for her. The message I gave was an important one — sometimes we just can't go ahead with plans but have to take care of ourselves.

The tests that I had taken the previous week confirmed the kidney stones. Now the decision was whether to have the easier lithotrip procedure, or full kidney surgery. It was felt that the lithotrip wouldn't do the job, and we decided on the surgery. The only problem was to find an operating room. We live in a world where it's a problem to find a place to park your car. I couldn't believe that it was equally difficult to find an operating room. I had come in on Monday, and between the doctors' schedules and the operating room schedule, I couldn't have the surgery until a week from Tuesday.

Then, to complicate matters, I developed a staph infection and started running a fever.

I was concerned that they would postpone the surgery even more. I did everything I could to fight the fever. I took the medications prescribed, I walked, I blew on the machine that cleared your lungs, I drank as much as I could, and I put the ice packs on my body. I had a wedding I wanted to attend. I felt if they operated on Tuesday, I would have a chance to go to the wedding the following Sunday. However, if the operation were postponed, there would be no way I could go.

Another problem that had emerged was that Dr. Labes, my gynecologist, had found a sizable lump on my breast. Though to me, it was starting to feel like too much, I was concerned that to others it would just sound repetitious. This is something we with chronic illnesses have to learn to understand. Each new episode is important to us, but it does start to get boring to others. I questioned even putting these experiences in the book. However, I was soon challenged to use the coping skills that I have talked about. The first week, I was so miserable that it was difficult to do more than just exist. I began to feel concerned that perhaps I had come across as too much of a pollyanna in my writing. I'm always saying, "You can do it. Just find a way." I realized then, the importance of telling all of you suffering with chronic illness that sometimes it is really very hard. There are times when you may want to just give up. I know, giving up was starting to look very tempting to me.

Fortunately, I soon realized that I was going to have to cope — "big-time." Once again I went to my book to review the coping mechanisms that I had written about. I started to use many of the skills that I have shared with you throughout this book. One coping skill that I found particularly helpful this time was to ask for what I needed. Often when people would ask what I needed I would just say, "Oh, nothing." Now I was very clear. I wanted phone calls ... I wanted someone there after surgery ... I wanted cards and good wishes. Yes, I could use help, and I was specific. I found my friends and family were pleased to know exactly what it was I wanted. Instead of burdening them, I was actually helping them. They felt much better doing something that they knew would be helpful.

To my relief the mammogram showed the lump to be just a cyst. The operation went as scheduled on Tuesday. But the fever persisted and I was unable to go to the wedding. We can learn to live with disappointments when we realize that the days ahead will bring other joys. Sometimes we just have to get through the present.

But the present wasn't so easy to get through. I now had developed excruciating pain in my leg and back. I was beginning to feel like a hypochondriac. There was no explanation for these pains but I was having a difficult time handling them. Pain medication wasn't even helping. I know many of you can identify with the time before you were diagnosed — a time when you were suffering but nobody knew why.

In spite of the pain "of unknown origin," after three weeks I went home from the hospital, because in the hospital I was growing weaker every day. I was unable to walk even to the bathroom. I felt that at home I would be encouraged to get back to more normal living, and regain my strength. The pain prevented this. I came home on a Friday and Saturday I mustered enough strength to go to the Greenbergs' party for a little while. It took an entire day just to get dressed, but it was nice to do something "normal."

By Sunday, it was impossible to take the IV. It was like torture. We did some detective work. We were able to identify the pain intensifying when the IV was running. This wasn't comforting because I was IV-dependent. Without the IVs, I would become dehydrated and go into kidney failure. When Dr.Bodzin realized that I couldn't take the IVs he arranged for me to go into surgery as an emergency. He called at 2:50 on Monday and told us to get to the hospital immediately. The operating room was scheduled for 3:30. Again we rushed over to the hospital. I had time to make one phone call and leave some instructions, and soon I was back in surgery.

Dr. Bodzin introduced me to the surgical team and said, "She's a very difficult patient." I raised my head from the surgical table and corrected him: "My body may be difficult, but I'm charming." Dr. Bodzin agreed, and I don't remember much after that. It was just a local anesthetic, but fortunately I slept through the whole operation. The goal was to find a vein for a new port so that I could have an access for my IVs. Later, Dr. Bodzin told me they tried to find a vein in my jugular and went in four times. He began to think that he wouldn't be able to save me and then the fifth time he got in. Needless to say, we were all very happy. A one in a million quirk had caused the IV line to leak and hit a nerve. Replacing it solved the "pain" problem.

The lessons I learned from this recent bout follow because I feel they are important for you as well:

- No matter how much has gone wrong, it may not be the end. And no matter how much we have prepared, there may be more to come.

- We will at times feel overwhelmed.

But using our coping skills, we can meet the challenge.

Audrey Kron
August, 1995

Dear Readers:

Now you have completed this book and the choice is yours. You can decide to take the information you have acquired and start taking steps to take control of your life and your illness, or you can procrastinate and wait for "someday" to do something. I think it is appropriate that I leave you with a poem entitled:

SomeDay I'll by Dennis Whatley

THERE IS AN ISLAND FANTASY
OF SOMEDAY ISLE I'LL NEVER SEE.
WHERE RECESSION STOPS, INFLATION CEASES,
OUR MORTGAGE IS PAID, OUR PAY INCREASES.

THAT SOMEDAY ISLE WHERE PROBLEMS END,
WHERE EVERY PIECE OF MAIL IS FROM A FRIEND.
WHERE THE CHILDREN ARE SWEET AND ALREADY GROWN,
WHERE ALL OTHER NATIONS CAN GO IT ALONE.

WHERE WE ALL RETIRE AT FORTY-ONE,
PLAYING BACKGAMMON IN THE ISLAND SUN.
MOST UNHAPPY PEOPLE LOOK TO TOMORROW
TO ERASE TODAY'S HARDSHIP AND SORROW.

THEY PUT HAPPINESS ON LAY-A-WAY
AND STRUGGLE THROUGH A BLUE TODAY.
BUT HAPPINESS CANNOT BE SOUGHT,
IT CAN'T BE EARNED, IT CAN'T BE BOUGHT.

cont'd...

LIFE'S MOST IMPORTANT REVELATION,
IS THAT THE JOURNEY MEANS MORE THAN THE DESTINATION.
HAPPINESS IS WHERE YOU ARE RIGHT NOW,
PUSHING A PENCIL OR PUSHING A PLOW,

GOING TO SCHOOL OR STANDING IN LINE,
WATCHING OR WAITING OR TASTING THE WINE.
IF YOU LIVE IN THE PAST, YOU'LL BECOME SENILE.
IF YOU LIVE IN THE FUTURE, YOU'RE ON SOMEDAY ISLE.

THE FEAR OF RESULTS IS PROCRASTINATION.
THE JOY OF TODAY IS CELEBRATION.
YOU CAN SAVE, YOU CAN SLAVE, TRUDGING MILE AFTER MILE,
BUT YOU'LL NEVER SET FOOT ON YOUR SOMEDAY ISLE.

WHEN YOU'VE PAID ALL YOUR DUES AND PUT IN YOUR TIME,
OUT OF NOWHERE COMES ANOTHER MOUNT EVEREST TO CLIMB.
FROM THIS DAY FORWARD, MAKE IT YOUR VOW,
TAKE SOMEDAY I'LL, AND MAKE IT YOUR NOW.

APPENDIX ONE
SUPPORT GROUPS

Aids
National Association of People with Aids
1413 K St. NW Seventh Floor
Washington, DC 20005-3442
(202) 898-0414 Fax: 202/898-0435
Web: http://www.thecure.org

Amyotrophic Lateral Sclerosis Association
21021 Ventura Blvd., #321
Woodland Hills, CA 91364
(818) 340-7500 (800) 782-4747 Fax: 818/ 340-2060
Web: http://www.alsa.org

Arthritis
Arthritis Foundation
1330 West Peachtree Street
Atlanta, GA 30309
(404) 872-7100 (800) 283-7800 Fax: 404/ 872-0457
Web: http://wwwarthritis.org

Asthma and Allergy Foundation of America
1125 Fifteenth Street, N.W. Suite 502
Washington, D.C. 20005
(202) 466-7643 (800) 7-ASTHMA Fax: 202/466-8940

Autoimmune Related Diseases
American Autoimmune Related Diseases Association
Michigan National Bank Building
15475 Gratiot Ave.
Detroit, MI 48205
(313) 371-8600 (800) 598-4668 Fax: 313/ 371-6002
E-Mail: aarda@aol.com

Cancer
American Cancer Society
1599 Clinton Road, N. E.
Atlanta, GA 30329
(404) 320-3333 (800) ACS-2345 Fax: 404/ 329-7530
Web: www.cancer.org

Cerebral Palsy
United Cerebral Palsy Association
1522 K Street N.W. Suite 1112
Washington, D.C. 20005
(800) 872-5287

Chronic Pain
American Chronic Pain Association
P.O. Box 850
Rocklin, CA 95677
(916) 632-0922 Fax: 916/ 632-3208
E-Mail: acpa@1x.netcom.com

Chronic Pain
National Chronic Pain Outreach Association, Inc.
7979 Old Georgetown Road # 100
Bethesda, MD 20814
(301) 652-4948 Fax: 301/907-0745
E-Mail: NCPOAI@AOL.COM

Cleft Palate
Cleft Palate Foundation
1218 Grandview Ave.
Pittsburgh, PA 15211
(800) 24-CLEFT Fax: 412/ 481-0847

Crohn's and Colitis Foundation of America, Inc.
386 Park Avenue South, 17th floor
New York, NY 10016-8804
(800) 932-2423 Fax: 212/ 779-4098
Web: http://www.ccfa.org
E-Mail: info@ ccfa.org

Cystic Fibrosis Foundation
6931 Arlington Rd.
Bethesda, MD 20814
(301) 951-4422 (800) 344-4823 Fax: 301/ 951-6378
Web: http://www.cff.org

Diabetes
American Diabetes Association
1660 Duke Street
Alexandria, VA 22314
(703) 549-1500 (800) 232-3472 Fax: 703/ 549-6995
Web: htpp://www.diabetes.org

Ehlers-Danlos National Foundation
P.O. Box 35177
Los Angeles, CA 90035
(213)651-3039 Fax: (213) 651-1366

Epilepsy Foundation of America
4351 Garden City Drive
Landover, MD 20785-2267
(800) 332-1000 (English & Spanish) 301-459-3700
Fax: 301/ 577-4941
Web: www.efa.org.

Facial Differences
About Face
(support and information organization dealing with facial differences)
P.O. Box 93
Limekiln, PA 19135
(800) 225-FACE Fax: 610/ 689-4479
E-Mail: abtface@aol.com
Canada:
99 Crowns Lane, 4th Floor
Toronto, Ont. (800) 665-FACE Fax: 416/ 944-2488
E-Mail: aface@10.org

Fatigue Syndrome & Fibromyalgia Association
National Chronic Fatigue Syndrome & Fibromyalgia Association Inc.
P.O. Box 18426
Kansas City, MO 64133
(816) 313-2000 (24 hours) Fax: 816/ 524-6782
KEAL 55A@PRODIGY.COM

Genetic Diseases
Alliance of Genetic Support Groups
35 Wisconsin Circle, Suite 440
Chevy Chase, MD 20815-7015
(301) 652-5553 (800) 336-GENE Fax: 301/ 654-0171
E-Mail: alliance@capaccess.org
Web: http://medhlp.netusa.net/www/agsg.htm

Graves Disease
National Graves Disease Foundation
Dr. Nancy Patterson
2 Tsitsi Ct.
Brevard, NC 28712
(704) 877- 5251

Headaches
Ache Headache Support Group
875 Kings Highway, Suite 200
Woodbury, NJ 08096-3172
(609) 845-0322 (800) 255-ACHE Fax: 609/ 384-5811
headquarters @ ache.ccmail.compuserve.com

Heart Disease
American Heart Association National Center
7272 Greenville Ave.
Dallas, TX 75231-4596
(800) 242-8721 (800) 553-6321 (Stroke Connection)
Fax: 214/ 696-5211
Web: http://www.amhrt.org

Hemophilia
National Hemophilia Foundation
(Other bleeding disorders including Von Willerand)
110 Greene Street, Suite 303
New York, NY 10012
(212) 219-8180
(800) 42-HANDI*
(*Hemophilia and Aids Network for Dissemination of Information)
Fax: 212/ 431-0906
Internet: www.infonhf.

Herpes
American Social Health Assoc.
Herpes Resource Center (HRC)
P.O. Box 13827
Research Triangle Park, NC 27709-9940
Fax: 919/361-8425
Web: http://sunsite.unc.edu/ASHA/

Huntington's Disease Society of America, Inc.
140 West 22nd Street 6th Floor
New York, N Y 10011-2420
(212) 242-1968 (800) 345-4372 Fax: 212/ 243-2443
Web: http:neuro-www2.mgh.harvard.edu/hdsa/hdsamain.nclk

Ichthyosis & Related Skin Types
F.I.R.S.T. (Foundation for Ichthyosis & Related Skin Types)
P.O. Box 20921
Raleigh, NC 27619-0921
(919) 782-5728 (800) 545-3286 Fax: 919/ 781-0679

Immune Deficiency Diseases
Immune Deficiency Foundation
25 West Chesapeake Avenue, Suite 206
Towson, MD 21204
410-321-6647 800-296-4433 Fax: 410/ 321-9165
Internet: http://www.clark.net/pub/idf/

Incontinence
National Association for Continence
P.O. Box 8310
Spartanburg , SC 29305-8310
800-BLADDER
(803) 579-7900 for SC Fax: 803/ 579-7902
Internet: www.nafc.org

Interstitial Cystitis
National Patient Support Network
Interstitial Cystitis Asoc. (ICA)
P.O. Box 1553
Madison Square Station
New York, N.Y. 10159

cont'd....

212-979-6057 800-HELPICA
Fax:212/677-6139
Web:http://www.ichelp.com

Kidney Disease
American Association of Kidney Patients
100 S. Ashley Drive, Suite 280
Tampa, FL 33602
(800) 749-2257 Fax: 813/ 223-0001
AOL: aakpnat@aol.com

Lupus Foundation of America, Inc.
1300 Piccard Suite 200
Rockville, MD 20850
(301) 670-9292 800-558-0121
Fax: 301/670-9486
Web: Living with Lupus
http://www.lupus.org/lupus

Lyme Disease
43 Winton Road
Brunswick, N. J. 08816
Fax: 908/238-8292

Multiple Sclerosis
National Multiple Sclerosis Society
733 Third Ave,
New York, NY 10017-3288
(212) 986-3240 (800) 344-4867 Fax: 212/ 986-7981
Web: http://www.nmss.org
E-Mail: NET2NMSS.ORG

Muscular Dystrophy Association
3300 Sunrise Drive
Tucson, AZ 85718
(520) 529-2000 (800) 572-1717 Fax: 520/ 529-5300
Web:http://www.mdausa.org.

Myasthenia Gravis Foundation of America, Inc.
222 S. Riverside Plaza, Suite 1540
Chicago IL 60606-9524
(312) 258-0522 (800) 541-5454 Fax: 312/ 258-0461
Web: http://www.med.unc.edu/mgfa/

Ostomy
United Ostomy Association (UOA)
36 Executive Park, Suite 120
Irvine, CA 92714
(800) 826-0826 (714) 660-8624 Fax: 714/ 660-9262
Web: http://www.gulf.net/civic/org/uoa

Parkinson's Disease
National Parkinson Foundation, Inc.
1501 N.W. Ninth Ave.
Miami, FL 33136-1494
(305) 547-6666 (800) 327-4545 Fax: 305/ 548-4403
Web: http://www.parkinson.org
E-Mail: mailbox@npf.med.miami.edu

Pseudo-Obstruction & Hirschsprung's Disease
American Pseudo-Obstruction & Hirschsprung's Disease Society
P.O. Box 772
Medford, MA 02155-0066
(617) 395-4255 Fax: 617/ 396-6868
Web: http://www.tiac.net/users/aphs

Psoriasis
National Psoriasis Foundation
6600 S.W. 92nd Ave. # 300
Portland, OR 97223
(503) 244-7404 (800) 723-9166
Fax: 503/ 245-0626
Web: http://www.psoriasis.org

Reflex Sympathetic Dystrophy Syndrome Association
116 Haddon Ave
Haddonfield, NJ 08033-2306
(609)795-8845(1:30-5pm) Fax:609/795-8845
Web:http://cyboarad.com/rsds

Scleroderma
United Scleroderma Foundation
P.O. Box 399 Watsonville, CA 95077
(408) 728-2202 (800) 722- HOPE Fax: 408/ 728-3328
Web: http://www.scleroderma.com/

Sickle Cell Disease Foundation
200 Corporate Pointe # 495
Culver City, CA 90230-7633
310-216-6363 800-421-8453 Fax: 310/215-3722

Sjogren's Syndrome
National Sjogren's Syndrome
P.O. Box 42207
Phoenix, ARIZ 85080
602-516-0787 Voice Mail: 800-395-6772
Fax: 602-516-0111
Web: http://www.sjogrens.org/
E-Mail: Nssa@aol.com

Spinal Cord Injury
National Spinal Cord Injury Association
8300 Colesville Road Suite 551
Silver Springs, MD 20910
301-588-6959 (800) 962-9629 Fax: 301/ 588-9414
Web: spinalcord.org.(as of Oct. 15, 1996)
E-Mail: NSCIA2@AOL.COM

Tay-Sachs and Allied Diseases
National Tay-Sachs and Allied Diseases Association
2001 Beacon Street
Brookline, MA 02146
(617) 277-4463 Fax: 617-277-0134
E-Mail: NTSAD-BOSTON@WORLDNET.ATT.NET

Tourette Syndrome Association, Inc.
42-40 Bell Boulevard
Bayside, NY 11361-2874
(718) 224-2999 800-237-0717 Fax: 718/ 279-9596
E-Mail:Tourette@1xnetcom/com

Tuberous Sclerosis
National Tuberous Sclerosis Association
8181 Professional Place, Suite 110
Landover, MD 20785
(301) 459-9888 (800) 225-6872 Fax: 301/459-0394
E-Mail: ntsa@aol.com

Tube-Feeding
Oley Foundation, Inc.
214 HUN Memorial
Albany Medical Center A-23
Albany, NY 12208
(518) 262-5079 800-776-6539 Fax:262-5528
Family PEN Network 800-776-6539

Well Spouse Foundation
610 Lexington Ave.,
New York, NY 10022-6005
212-644-1241 (800) 838-0879 Fax: 212/ 644-1338
E-Mail: wellspouse@aol.com.

If you are having a problem locating a support group for your illness you might try:

Rare Disorders
National Organization for Rare Disorders, Inc.
P.O. Box 8923
New Fairfield, CT 06812-8923
(203) 746-6518 (800) 999-6673 Fax: 203/746-6481

If you still have not been able to find your organization, call the American Self-Help Clearinghouse. They will either give you the number, or if an organization for your illness doesn't exist, they will help you form one. Their number is as follows:

American Self-Help Clearinghouse
Northwest Covenant Medical Center
25 Pocono Rd.
Denville, N J 07834
(201) 625-7101 Fax: 201/ 625-8848
Web:http://www.cmhc.com/selfhelp/
E-Mail:ASHC@bc/cybernex.net

APPENDIX TWO
READINGS

BOOKS ON CHRONIC ILLNESS

Carter, Rosalynn, *Helping Yourself Help Others: A Book for Caregivers.* Times Books/Random House, New York, 1994.

Caudill, M.D., Ph.D., Margaret *Managing Pain before It Manages You.* The Guilford Press, New York, 1995.

Cousins, Norman, *Anatomy of an Illness.* Norton Publishing, New York, 1979.

Donoghue, Paul J., Ph.D., and Siegel, Mary E., Ph.D., *Sick and Tired of Feeling Sick and Tired.* W.W. Norton & Co., New York, 1993.

Jacobs, Pamela D., M. A., *500 Tips for Coping With Chronic Illness.* Robert D. Reed Publishers, San Francisco, 750 LaPlaya, Suite 647 S.F., CA 94121, 1995.

Hanner, Linda and Witek, John.J., M.D. and Clift, Robert, Ph.D., *When You're Sick and Don't Know Why: Coping with your Undiagnosed Illness.* D.C.I. Publishing, P.O. Box 47945, Minneapolis, MN 55447-972, 1991.

Kievman, Beverly with Blackmun, Susie, *For Better or Worse, A Couple's Guide to Dealing with Chronic Illness.* Contemporary Books, 180 North Michigan Ave, Chicago, IL 60601, 1989.

Kobrin Pitzele, Sefra, *We are Not Alone—Learning to Live with Chronic Illness.* Workman Publishing, New York, 1985.

Mies, Monica Loose, *Home Care for the Chronically Ill or Disabled Child.* Harper & Row, New York, 1985.

Polin, Irene, and Golant, S.R., *Taking Charge: Overcoming the Challenges of Long-Term Illness.* Times Book, Random House, New York, 1994.

Register, Cheri, *Living with Chronic Illness—Days of Patience and Passion.* The Free Press, A Division of Macmillan Inc., New York, 1987.

Weiss, Louise, *Access to the World, A Travel Guide for the Handicapped.* Henry Holt and Company, New York, 1986.

Wheeler, Eugenie G. and Dace-Lombard, Joyce *Living Creatively with Chronic Illness.* Pathfinder Publishing, Ventura, CA 1989.

BOOKS ON THE MIND-BODY CONNECTION, STRESS, AND MEDITATION.

Benson, Herbert, M.D., *The Relaxation Response.* Morrow, New York, 1975.

Borysenko, Joan, Ph.D., *Minding the Body, Minding the Mind.* Bantam Books, New York, 1988.
Guilt is the Teacher, Love is the Lesson. Warner Books, New York, 1990.

Chopra, Deepak, M.D., *Ageless Body, Timeless Mind.* Harmony Books, New York, 1993.

Cousins, Norman, *Head First, the Biology of Hope.* E.P. Dutton, New York, 1989.

Hay, Louise L, *You Can Heal Your Life.* Hay House, Santa Monica, CA, 1984.

Kabat-Zinn, Jon, Ph.D., *Full Catastrophe Living.* Delacorte Press, New York, 1990.

Locke, Steven, M.D. and Colligan, Douglas, *The Healer Within*. E.P. Dutton, New York, 1986.

Miller, Lyle H., Ph.D. and Smith, Alma Dell, *The Stress Solution*. Pocket Books, New York, 1993.

Moyers, Bill, *Healing and The Mind*. Doubleday, New York, 1993.

Ornstein, Robert, Ph.D., and Sobel, David, M.D., *Healthy Pleasures*. Addison Wesley Publishing Co., Inc., Reading, Mass., 1989.

Pearsall, Paul, Ph.D., *Super Immunity*. McGraw-Hill, New York, 1987. *The Pleasure Principle: Discovering a New Way to Health.* A Nightingale Conant Tape, 800-323-5552.

Pelletier, Kenneth R., Ph.D., *Mind as Healer Mind as Slayer*. Dell Publishing, New York, 1977.

Siegel, Bernie, M.D., *Love, Medicine and Miracles.* Harper & Row, New York. 1986. *Peace, Love and Healing*. Harper & Row, New York, 1989.

BOOKS ON RELATIONSHIPS

Bach, George R., Ph.D., and Wyden, Peter, *The Intimate Enemy: How to Fight Fair in Love and Marriage*. Avon, New York, 1970.

Bradshaw, John, *Homecoming: Reclaiming and Championing Your Inner Child*. Bantam Books, New York, 1990.

Bramson, Robert M., Ph.D., *Coping with Difficult People—in Business and In Life.* Ballentine Books, a division of Random House, New York, 1981.

Branden, Nathaniel Ph.D., *6 Pillars of Self Esteem*. Bantam, New York, 1994.

Bugen, Larry A., Ph.D., *Love and Renewal.* New Harbinger Publications, Inc., 1990. (5674 Shattuck Ave, Oakland, CA 94609)

Carnegie, Dale, *How to Win Friends and Influence People.* Simon and Schuster, New York, 1981.

Ellenberg, Daniel, Ph.D., and Bell, Judith, M.S., M.F.C.C., *Lovers for Life.* Aslan Publishing, Santa Rosa, CA, 3356 Coffey Lane, Santa Rosa, CA, 95403, 1995.

Gray, John, Ph.D., *Men are from Mars, Women are from Venus*. Harper-Collins Publishers, Inc., New York, 1992.

Hendrix, Harville, Ph.D., *Getting the Love You Want.* Henry Holt & Co., New York, 1988.

Kleveer, Phil, *Are we Having Fun Yet*? International Marriage Encounter, St. Paul, MN, 1988.

Love, Patricia, Ph.D., Robinson, J. O., *Hot Monogamy* Penguin Books, New York, 1994.

Louden, Jennifer, *The Couple's Comfort Book: A Creative Guide for Renewing Passion, Pleasure & Commitment*. Harper, San Francisco, CA 1994.

Matthews, Andrew, *Making Friends: A Guide to Getting Along with People*. Price Stern Sloan, Inc., 1150 Olympic Blvd., Suite 650, L.A, CA 90064, 1991.

Markman, Howard, Stanley, Scott and Blumberg, Susan, *Fighting for Your Marriage.* Jossey-Bass Publishers, San Francisco, CA 1994.

Pearsall, Paul, Ph.D., *Super Marital Sex*. Doubleday, New York, 1987.

Scarf, Maggie, *Intimate Partners.* Random House, New York, 1987.

Tannen, Deborah, Ph.D., *You Just Don't Understand.* William Morrow and Co. Inc., New York, 1990.

Young-Eisendrath, Polly, Ph.D., *You're Not What I Expected: Breaking the 'He said-She-said' Cycle.* Simon & Schuster, New York, 1993.

BOOKS ON IMPROVING THE QUALITY OF YOUR LIFE

Beattie, Melody, *Codependent No More: How to Stop Controlling Others and Start Caring for Yourself.* Harper & Row, San Francisco, CA, 1987.

Burns, David, M.D., *Feeling Good: The New Mood Therapy.* Penguin, New York, 1980.

Elgin, Suzette Haden, *The Gentle Art of Verbal Self Defense.* Dorset Press, a division of Marboro Books Corp., 1980.

Fensterhein, Herbert, Ph.D., and Baer, Jean, *Don't Say Yes When You Want to Say No.* Dell Publishing Co., New York, 1975.

Jakubowski, Patricia and Lange, Arthur J., *The Assertive Option.* Research Press Co., Champaign, IL, 1978.

Lerner, Harriet Goldhor, Ph.D., *The Dance of Anger.* Harper & Row, New York, 1985.

Mackenzie, Alec, *The Time Trap.* AMACOM, a division of American Management Association, 135 West 50th Street, New York 10020, 1990.

Matthews, Andrew, *Being Happy.* Price Stern Sloan, Inc., L.A., 11150 Olympic Blvd. Suite 650, Los Angeles, CA 90064, 1990.

McGrath, Ph.D., and Fanning, Patrick, *Self-Esteem: A Proven Program of Cognitive Techniques for Assessing, Improving and Maintaining your Self-Esteem*. New Harbinger Publications, Inc., Oakland, CA, 1992.

McWilliams, Peter, *You Can't Afford The Luxury of A Negative Thought: A Book for People with Any Life-Threatening Illness—Including Life.* Prelude Press, L.A., CA, 1995. (8159 Santa Monica Blvd., L.A. 90046). *Do It! Let's Get Off Our Buts* Prelude Press, Los Angeles, CA, 1991.

Simon, Sidney B., Ph.D., and Suzanne, *Forgiveness.* Warner Books, New York, 1990.

Smith, Ann W., M.S., *Overcoming Perfectionism, The Super Human Syndrome*. Health Communications, Deerfield Beach, FL 1990.

Smith, M. J., *When I Say No, I Feel Guilty.* Bantam Books, New York, 1975.

GENERAL INSPIRATIONAL BOOKS

Buscaglia, Leo, Ph.D., *Living, Loving & Learning*. Fawcett Columbine, New York, 1982.

Canfield, Jack and Hansen, Mark Victor, *Chicken Soup for the Soul: 101 Stories to Open the Heart and Rekindle the Spirit.* Health Communications, Inc., 3201 S.W. 15th St., Deerfield Beach, FL 33442-8190, 1993.

Cheng, Nien, *Life and Death in Shanghai*. Penguin Books, New York, 1986.

Cramer, Kathryn D., *Staying on Top When Your World is Upside Down*. Viking Penguin, New York, 1990.

Frankl, Viktor E., *Man's Search for Meaning.* Washington Square Press, New York, 1959.

Kushner, Harold S., *When Bad Things Happen to Good People.* Avon Books, New York, 1983.

Pearsall, Paul, Ph.D., *Making Miracles.* Prentice Hall Press, New York, 1991.

Segal, Julius, M.D., *Winning Life's Toughest Battles.* McGraw-Hill, New York, 1986.

BOOKS ON PARENTING

Finston, Peggy, M.D., *Parenting Plus—Raising Children With Special Health Needs.* Dutton, New York, 1990.

Gordon, Dr. Thomas, *P.E.T. Parent Effectiveness Training.* Peter H. Wyden, Inc. New York, 1988.

Wolf, Anthony E. Ph.D., *Get Out of My Life, but First Could You Drive Me and Cheryl to the Mall? - A Parent's Guide to the New Teenager.* The Noonday Press (a division of Farrar, Straus and Giroux, 19 Union Square West, New York, 10003), 1991.

BOOKS ON HUMOR

Assimov, Isaac, *Treasury of Humor: 640 Jokes, Anecdotes and Limericks.* Houghton Mifflen Company, Boston, 1971.

Bombeck, Erma, *All I Know About Animal Behavior I Learned in Loehman's Dressing Room.* Harper Collins, New York, 1995.

continued...

Brilliant Ashleigh, *I May not be Totally Perfect but Parts of Me are Excellent.* Woodbridge Press Publishing Co., Santa Barbara, CA 93111, 1979. *I Try to Take One Day at a Time: But Sometimes Several Days Attack Me at Once.* Woodbridge Press Publishing Co. P.O. Box 209, Santa Barbara, CA 93102, 1987.

Green, Lila, *Making Sense of Humor: How to Add Joy to* Your *Life.* Knowledge, Ideas and Trends, Inc. 1131 Tolland Turnpike, Suite 175, Manchester, CT 060401, 1994.

Guisewite, Cathy, *Reflections, A Cathy Collection.* Andrews and Mc Meel, A Universal Press Syndicate Co., Kansas City, MO 1991.

Mason, Eileen, *Great Book of Funny Quotes, Witty Words for Every Day of the Year.* Sterling Publishing Co., Inc., New York, 1993.

Schultz, Charles M., *Around the World in 45 Years—Charlie Brown's Anniversary Celebration.* Andrews and Mc Neel, A Universal Press Syndicate Company, Kansas City, MO 1994.

Watterson, Bill, *The Calvin and Hobbes Tenth Anniversary Book.* Andrews & Mc Neel, Kansas City, MO 1995.

Notes:

Notes:

Notes:

To obtain additional copies, or to communicate with the author, contact:

Audrey Kron
Center for Coping with Chronic Illness
7466 Pebble Lane
West Bloomfield, MI 48322-3521
phone: 248-626-6960 fax: 248-626-1379

The price of the book is $16. (Canadian funds: $21.)
When ordering, add $3 for shipping and handling.
Discounts on orders of 10 or more copies are available.

Contact the author if your organization is interested in sponsoring the sale of the book in exchange for a share of the proceeds.

To order copies of *Meeting the Challenge*, send the completed form to:

Audrey Kron, M.A.,
Center for Coping with Chronic Illness,
7466 Pebble Lane,
West Bloomfield, MI 48322-3521

Name: ____________________
Address:: ____________________
____________________ Zip ____________
Phone: ____________________ Fax: ____________

Send this book as a gift to:

Name: ____________________
Address:: ____________________
____________________ Zip ____________
Phone: ____________________ Fax: ____________

Please send ______ books @ $16.00 each : ____________
(Canadian funds: $21.00)
Add: Shipping and handling @ $3.00 each ____________

Total: *(check is enclosed)* ____________

How did you learn about this book? ____________________
____
____

for quantity orders please call for special prices.
Audrey Kron: 248-626-6960 fax: 248-626-1379